Study Guide for

Introduction to Human Anatomy and Physiology

Fourth Edition

Revised Reprint

Lois A. Ball, PhD
Science and Education Consultant
Adjunct Professor
Honors College, University of South Florida

ELSEVIER

ELSEVIER

3251 Riverport Lane
Maryland Heights, MO 63043

STUDY GUIDE FOR INTRODUCTION TO HUMAN ANATOMY
AND PHYSIOLOGY - REVISED REPRINT

ISBN: 978-0-323-53123-8

Notice

Executive Content Strategist: Kellie White
Content Development Manager: Billie Sharp
Content Development Specialist: Heather Yocum
Publishing Services Manager: Hemamalini Rajendrababu
Project Manager: Sukanthi Sukumar
Cover Designer: Gopalakrishnan Venkataraman

Printed in the United States of America

Last digit is the print number: 9 8 7 6

Using Your Study Guide

Learning about the sciences of human anatomy and physiology - understanding the construction and functions of the body - provides an essential foundation for a career in health sciences and related fields. The varied exercises, labeling diagrams, thought-provoking questions, and puzzles presented herein are designed to help you understand and integrate the words and concepts presented in the textbook, *Introduction to Human Anatomy and Physiology*, by Eldra Pearl Solomon, PhD. Reading the textbook and completing the corresponding study guide materials together, as each chapter is presented, will help you gain knowledge and confidence in the subject matter.

The following steps will guide your learning experience with this Study Guide.

1. Read the Chapter Guide presented at the beginning of the chapter. The chapter guide reflects the organization of the corresponding textbook chapter and provides you with an overview of the material in the Study Guide chapter.

2. Read the Learning Objectives and refer back to them frequently as you work through each part of the chapter. The Learning Objectives tell you what you need to do to demonstrate mastery of the material.

3. Complete the **Learn the Terms** questions for each section in Part 1. Answers are available to instructors on Evolve. Reread parts of the textbook to correct and learn misunderstood words and concepts.

4. Label the diagrams that are provided in **Learn the Terms** Part 1 of the Study Guide. Then check the accuracy of your labels by consulting the corresponding labeled diagram presented in the textbook.

5. When you feel confident that you have learned the material in the chapter you are studying, check your level of mastery by completing **Assess Your Understanding** in Part 2 of the chapter. Answers are available for instructors on Evolve.

6. To further build your confidence and apply your new understanding, answer Part 3 - **Accept the Challenge** questions and complete **The Puzzle**, a crossword or search-and-find puzzle at the end of each chapter. Answers and puzzle solutions are available for instructors on Evolve.

Contents

1 Introducing the Human Body

CHAPTER GUIDE

I. Just what are anatomy and physiology?
II. The body has several levels of organization
III. Ions, inorganic compounds, and organic compounds interact
    A. Acids, bases, and salts dissociate into ions
    B. Organic compounds are more complex than inorganic compounds
IV. Metabolism is essential to maintenance, growth, and repair of the body
V. Homeostatic mechanisms maintain an appropriate internal environment
    A. Negative feedback systems restore homeostasis
    B. Positive feedback systems intensify a changing condition

VI. The body has a basic plan
    A. Directional terms for the body are relative
    B. The body has three main planes
    C. We can identify specific body regions
    D. There are two main body cavities
    E. It is important to view the body as a whole

LEARNING OBJECTIVES

1. Define anatomy and physiology, and explain why these disciplines are considered sciences.
2. Identify and briefly describe the levels of biological organization in the body, from the simplest (the chemical level) to the most complex (the organism).
3. Briefly describe the principal organ systems and summarize the functions of each.
4. Contrast ions, inorganic compounds, and organic compounds; briefly describe four important groups of organic compounds.
5. Define metabolism, and contrast anabolism and catabolism.
6. Define homeostasis, and contrast negative and positive feedback mechanisms.
7. Describe the anatomical positions of the body.
8. Define and apply the principal directional terms used in anatomy.
9. Identify sagittal, transverse, and frontal sections of the body and body structures.
10. Define and locate the principal regions and cavities of the body.

PART 1: LEARN THE TERMS

Match the following terms to the correct definitions by writing the corresponding letter in the space provided. (Section I)

| A. anatomy | B. cell biology | C. dissection | D. endocrinology | E. gross anatomy |
| F. histology | G. immunology | H. microscopic anatomy | I. neurophysiology | J. physiology |

1. _____ focuses on structures that can be studied by dissection

2. _____ branch of science that studies body function

3. _____ study of tissues

4. _____ focuses on structures that must be studied with microscopes

5. _____ branch of science that studies body structure

6. _____ study of the structure, function, and interaction of cells

7. _____ study of the body's defense system

8. _____ focuses on the functions of the nervous system

9. _____ study of hormones and the glands that produce them

10. _____ carefully cutting apart a body structure

Fill in the blank with the correct answer for each science statement. (Section I)

11. _____ is a way of thinking and a method of investigating the world in a systematic manner.

12. Science uses a series of steps called the _____ to investigate something of interest.

13. A researcher develops a tentative explanation, or _____, which can be tested.

14. A(n) _____ is performed to test the hypothesis.

15. A pharmaceutical company is testing a new medication. The _____ group receives the drug during the experiment.

16. The _____ group receives a placebo during the experiment.

17. A researcher does not know which group has received the drug to avoid _____.

18. A group of related hypotheses may eventually be considered a _____ if their experimental results are consistent.

Arrange the levels of biological organization in the body from simplest to most complex, and then unscramble the circled letters to correctly complete the final sentence. (Section II)

19. ◯ _ _ _ _ _ _ _ ◯

20. _ _ ◯ _ ◯ _ _ _ _

21. _ _ _ _ _ ◯

22. ◯ _ _ _ _ _

23. _ _ _ _ _   ◯ _ _ _ ◯ _

24. _ _ _ _ _ _ _ ◯

25. Atoms can combine chemically to form _ _ _ _ _ _ _ _ _.

Match the following terms to the correct definitions by writing the corresponding letter in the space provided. (Section III)

A. acid   **B. anion**   **C. base**   **D. cation**   **E. chemical compound**
F. electrolyte   **G. inorganic compound**   **H. ion**   **I. organic compound**   **J. pH**

26. _____ small, simple compounds such as water, salts, simple acids, and simple bases

27. _____ positively charged ion

28. _____ dissociates in solution to produce hydrogen ions (H^+) and some type of anion

29. _____ electrically charged atom or group of atoms

30. _____ substance that dissociates into ions when dissolved in water

31. _____ negatively charged ion

32. _____ dissociates in solution to produce hydroxide ions (OH⁻) and some cation

33. _____ large, complex compounds containing carbon

34. _____ molecule that consists of two or more different elements combined in a fixed proportion

35. _____ degree of a solution's acidity

Match the term on the left to the correct selection on the right. (Section III)

36. _____ carbohydrate   A. simple sugar that is the main source of energy for the body

37. _____ glucose   B. group of organic compounds containing fats and phospholipids

38. _____ glycogen   C. contains the instructions for making all the proteins needed by a cell

39. _____ lipid   D. large, complex molecules composed of subunits called amino acids

40. _____ fat   E. sugars and starches

41. _____ protein   F. protein catalysts that regulate chemical reactions

42. _____ amino acid   G. nucleic acid that is important for manufacturing proteins

43. _____ enzyme   H. carbohydrate with long, linked glucose chains

44. _____ DNA   I. type of lipid that stores energy

45. _____ RNA   J. subunits that make up proteins

Fill in the space to correctly complete each sentence. (Section IV)

46. Cells capture energy stored in glucose and other nutrient molecules in the breaking-down phase of metabolism called _____.

47. Energy released from nutrients is stored as _____, a special energy-storage compound.

48. _____ is all the interaction of chemical processes that take place within the body.

49. Cells obtain energy from nutrient molecules during a complex series of catabolic chemical reactions referred to as _____.

50. _____ is the building, or synthetic, phase of metabolism.

Match the following terms to the correct definitions by writing the corresponding letter in the space provided. (Section V)

A. negative feedback system   **B. positive feedback system**   **C. homeostatic mechanisms**
D. stressor   **E. homeostasis**

51. _____ variation from the steady state that sets off a series of events that intensify the changes

52. _____ change in some steady state triggers a response that is opposite to the change

53. _____ self-regulating control systems that maintain the body's steady state

54. _____ an appropriate internal environment, or steady state, for the body

55. _____ stimulus that disrupts homeostasis and causes stress in the body

Chapter **1** **Introducing the Human Body**

Match the term on the left to the correct selection on the right. (Section VI)

56. _____ bilateral symmetry   A. structures located toward the surface

57. _____ cranium   B. closer to the midline of the body

58. _____ vertebral column   C. toward the top of the head, or cranial

59. _____ anatomical position   D. front surface of the body, or ventral

60. _____ superior   E. toward one side of the body

61. _____ inferior   F. standing erect; eyes forward; arms at sides; palms/toes forward

62. _____ anterior   G. brain case

63. _____ posterior   H. closer to the body midline or point of attachment to the trunk

64. _____ medial   I. located away from the body surface

65. _____ lateral   J. toward the soles of the feet, or caudal

66. _____ proximal   K. farther from the midline or point of attachment to the trunk

67. _____ distal   L. back surface of the body, or dorsal

68. _____ superficial   M. right and left halves are mirror images

69. _____ deep   N. backbone

Unscramble the names of the three main planes and match them to their definition. (Section VI)

70. _____ tlfonra   divides the body into right and left parts, or mirror images

71. _____ evstarnres   divides the body into anterior and posterior parts

72. _____ atlasigt   divides the body into superior and inferior parts

Fill in the space to correctly complete each sentence. (Section VI)

73. Body cavities contain internal organs, also called _____.

74. The _____ and the _____ are the two principal body cavities.

75. The dorsal cavity is subdivided into the _____, which holds the brain, and the _____, which contains the spinal cord.

76. The ventral cavity is subdivided into the _____ and the _____, which are separated by a broad muscle called the _____.

77. The thoracic cavity consists of the _____, each containing a lung, and the _____, which contains the heart, thymus gland, and parts of the esophagus and trachea.

78. The heart is further surrounded by the _____.

79. The _____ is the upper portion of the abdominopelvic cavity, whereas the lower portion is the _____.

80. Males have an outpocket of the pelvic cavity, called the _____, which holds the testes.

81. Use answers from questions 73 through 80 to label Figure 1-1.

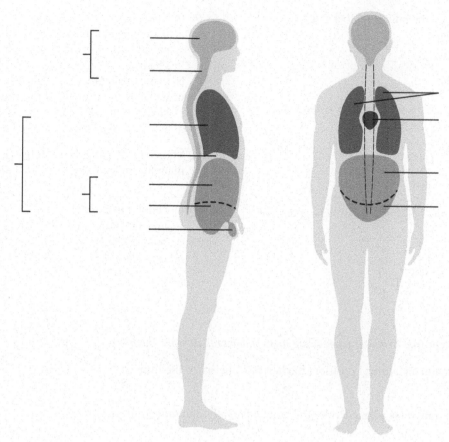

Figure 1-1

PART 2: ASSESS YOUR UNDERSTANDING

Select the correct answer.

1. Anatomy is the study of
   a. body function
   b. the nervous system
   c. body structure
   d. cell function

2. A physiologist studies
   a. the science of body function
   b. the respiratory system
   c. the science of body structure
   d. the physical sciences

3. A researcher tests a hypothesis by
   a. observation
   b. experimentation
   c. development
   d. investigation

4. The body's biological levels of organization, from simplest to most complex, are
   a. tissue, cellular, chemical, organ, organ system, organism
   b. chemical, cellular, tissue, organ, organ system, organism
   c. organism, organ, organ system, tissue, cellular, chemical
   d. chemical, cellular, organ, tissue, organ system, organism

5. A(n) _____ is an electrically charged atom or group of atoms.
   a. anion
   b. cation
   c. ion
   d. molecule

6. Amino acids are the building blocks of
   a. carbohydrates
   b. sugars
   c. lipids
   d. proteins

7. _____, a simple sugar, is the main source of energy for the body.
   a. glycogen
   b. protein
   c. nucleic acid
   d. glucose

8. Anabolism is the building, or synthetic, phase of

   _____
   a. catabolism
   b. cellular respiration
   c. metabolism
   d. homeostasis

9. In a positive feedback system,
   a. a change in a condition that varies from the steady state sets off events, which intensify the change.
   b. a stressor inhibits a response.
   c. a change in a condition that varies from the steady state triggers an opposite response.
   d. homeostasis is maintained by a variable stressor.

10. Metabolic activities are carefully regulated to maintain an appropriate internal environment, or

    _____
    a. cellular respiration
    b. metabolism
    c. homeostasis
    d. anabolism

Mark each statement true or false; correct the false statements to make them true.

11. _____ When in anatomical position, the heart is superior to the liver.

12. _____ The transverse plane divides the body bilaterally into mirror images.

13. _____ Humans are classified as vertebrates because they have a cranium and a vertebral column.

14. _____ The ankle is distal to the knee but proximal to the toes.

15. _____ The appendicular part of the body consists of the thorax, abdomen, and pelvis.

16. _____ The inguinal region of the body is the part of the lower extremity between the hip and the knee.

17. _____ The diaphragm separates the abdominal cavity and the pelvic cavity.

18. _____ The four quadrants of the abdominopelvic cavity are established by a midsagittal and a transverse plane that pass through the umbilicus.

19. _____ The pelvic cavity holds the urinary bladder, part of the large intestine, and male or female reproductive organs.

20. _____ The abdominopelvic cavity can be divided into nine regions using two transverse and two sagittal planes.

PART 3: ACCEPT THE CHALLENGE

1. Your blood pH is normally maintained at 7.4. Imagine that after exercising your blood becomes more acidic. Would a positive or negative feedback system return the blood pH to its normal state? Explain.

2. Why would a radiology technician need to understand human physiology in addition to anatomy?

3. Which division system of the abdominopelvic cavity, four quadrants or nine regions, would have greater specificity for identifying a particular location? Why?

4. Why is it important to view the body as a whole?

THE PUZZLE

Answer the questions to complete the crossword puzzle. (Refer to Table 1-2 for help.)

Organs and Organ Systems

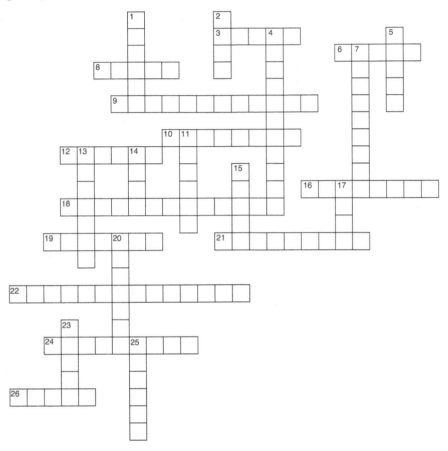

Across

3. female reproductive organ
6. heart pumps it throughout the body
8. starting point of digestive system
9. system responsible for procreation
10. system that supports and protects body
12. moves skeleton
16. system that moves parts of skeleton, pumps blood, and moves materials in body
18. system that provides protective covering for body
19. endocrine gland
21. system that works with nervous system to regulate metabolic activities
22. system that transports nutrients, gases, and hormones
24. system that ingests and digests foods; absorbs nutrients into blood
26. organ responsible for pumping blood

Down

1. also called lymphatic system; defends body against disease organisms and viruses
2. a component of the skeletal system
4. system that exchanges gas between blood and external environment
5. where two bones meet and move
7. system that collects and transports tissue fluid to blood
11. urinary system organ that excretes metabolic waste
13. system that excretes metabolic wastes; helps regulate volume and composition of blood
14. contained in a pleural cavity
15. nervous system organ
17. largest body organ
20. principal regulatory system; receives stimuli and transmits impulses
23. large digestive organ inferior to the lungs
25. male reproductive organs

2 Cells and Tissues

I. Cells are the living building blocks of the body
    A. Membranes surround the cell and divide it into compartments
    B. The nucleus controls cell activities
    C. The cytoplasm contains many types of organelles
II. Materials move through the plasma membrane by both passive and active processes
    A. Passive transport does not require the cell to expend metabolic energy
    B. Active transport requires metabolic energy

III. Cells communicate by signaling one another
IV. Cells divide by mitosis, producing genetically identical cells
V. Tissues are the fabric of the body
    A. Epithelial tissue protects the body
    B. Connective tissue joins body structures
    C. Muscle tissue is specialized to contract
    D. Nervous tissue controls muscles and glands
VI. Membranes cover or line body surfaces

LEARNING OBJECTIVES

1. Describe the general characteristics of cells.
2. State three functions of cell membranes and describe the structure of the plasma membrane.
3. Describe the structure and functions of the cell nucleus.
4. Describe, locate, and list the functions of the principal cytoplasmic organelles and be able to label them on a diagram.
5. Contrast passive transport with active transport of materials through cell membranes.
6. Predict whether cells will swell or shrink under different osmotic conditions.
7. Describe the events that take place in cell signaling.
8. Describe the stages of a cell's life cycle and summarize the significance of mitosis with respect to maintaining a constant chromosome number.
9. Describe the structure and functions of the principal types of tissues.
10. Contrast epithelial tissue with connective tissue.
11. Compare the three types of muscle tissue.
12. Contrast mucous membranes with serous membranes.

PART 1: LEARN THE TERMS

Match the following terms to the correct definitions by writing the corresponding letter in the space provided. (Section I)

A. chromosomes   B. cytoplasm   C. DNA   D. genes   E. genome
F. nuclear envelope   G. nucleus   H. organelles   I. phospholipids   J. plasma membrane

1. _____ control center of the cell

2. _____ surrounds and protects cell; regulates passage of materials into and out of cell

3. _____ jellylike material of the cell

4. _____ rod-shaped bodies made up of chromatin

5. _____ double membrane surrounding nucleus

6. _____ specialized structures scattered throughout the cell

7. _____ complete set of genes

8. _____ lipids that contain phosphorous

9. _____ chemical compound that makes up genes

10. _____ units of hereditary information governing cell structure and activity

Fill in the blank with the correct answer for each statement. (Section I)

11. The _____ is a granular region within the nucleus that assembles ribosomes.

12. The complex tunnel system made of membranes that extends throughout the cytoplasm is the _____.

13. _____ are organelles that function as factories to manufacture proteins.

14. Bacteria and foreign matter are destroyed by digestive enzymes contained in little sacs called _____.

15. The _____ processes and packages proteins.

16. A _____ is a small membrane-enclosed structure that holds or transports cargo within the cell.

17. A _____ is a membrane-enclosed sac, which forms around large ingested particles that enter the cell.

18. _____ are power plants within cells that perform cellular respiration.

19. The _____ is a dense network of protein filaments that provides structural support and aids in transportation of materials for the cell.

20. _____ are tiny hollow tubes that provide support to the cell.

21. Tiny hairlike organelles that project from the surface of some cells and move materials out of the cell are called _____.

22. A sperm cell has a whip-like tail called a _____ that propels it toward an ovum.

Match the term on the left to the correct selection on the right. (Section II)

23. _____ diffusion	A.	active transport in which a cell ingests food or bacteria
24. _____ osmosis	B.	cell uses stored energy to move materials against a concentration gradient
25. _____ isotonic	C.	diffusion of water molecules through a selectively permeable membrane
26. _____ hypertonic	D.	active transport in which folds of plasma membrane trap drops of fluid
27. _____ hypotonic	E.	solution with solute concentration equal to that of a cell
28. _____ filtration	F.	force in which solutes in a more concentrated solution pull water molecules across a membrane
29. _____ active transport	G.	solution with solute concentration less than that of cell
30. _____ phagocytosis	H.	net movement of molecules down a concentration gradient
31. _____ osmotic pressure	I.	solution with solute concentration more than that of a cell
32. _____ pinocytosis	J.	passage of material through membranes by mechanical pressure

Fill in the blanks to complete each sequential step of the cell signaling process, and then unscramble the circled letters to correctly complete the final sentence. (Section III)

33. Cells communicate by sending _ ◯ _ _ _ _ _ .

34. _ _ _ _ ◯ _ _ _ _ _ ◯ receive the signal in a process called _ _ _ _ _ _ _ _ _ _ _ .

35. The signal molecules may bind to a _ ◯ _ _ _ _ _ _ on the surface of the target cells.

36. In the process of _ _ _ _ ◯ _ _ _ _ _ _ ◯ _ _ _ _ _ , a receptor converts a signal outside of the cell to a signal inside of the cell that affects a cellular process.

37. The final process, _ _ ◯ _ _ _ _ _ , occurs when the cell responds to a signal by changing some activity.

38. Cell signaling helps to protect the body against invading _ _ _ _ _ _ _ _ organisms.

Match the following terms to the correct definitions by writing the corresponding letter in the space provided. (Section IV)

A. anaphase	**B. centrioles**	**C. centromere**	**D. interphase**	**E. meiosis**
F. metaphase	**G. mitosis**	**H. prophase**	**I. sister chromatids**	**J. telophase**

39. _____ cell nucleus divides and complete sets of chromosomes move to each end of the cell

40. _____ sister chromatids separate and become independent chromosomes

41. _____ chromosome begins to uncoil and disperse; spindles disappear

42. _____ constricted region of each chromosome

43. _____ chromatids are positioned along equator of cell; spindles attach to centromere

44. _____ duplicated chromosome pairs

45. _____ chromatin coils tightly forming dark, X-shaped bodies

46. _____ number of chromosomes in developing sperm and ova are halved

47. _____ cylindrical organelles composed of microtubules

48. _____ period between mitoses; cell makes new materials and grows

Fill in the blank with the correct answer for each statement. (Section V)

49. _____ is the microscopic study of _____; groups of closely associated cells that work together to perform a specific function or group of functions.

50. _____ protects the body by covering all free surfaces and lining cavities.

51. Cells of _____ epithelium are thin and flattened, whereas _____ epithelium consists of short cylinders, or cube-shaped cells.

52. _____ epithelial can appear hexagonal in a cross-section and may contain cilia that move materials over the tissue surface.

53. A gland consists of one or more epithelial cells specialized to produce and secrete products such as

_____, _____, _____, _____, or _____.

54. _____ glands have _____ and most of them are multicellular.

55. _____ glands do not have ducts; they release _____ into surrounding tissue fluid.

Chapter **2 Cells and Tissues**

56. _____ tissues join other body tissues and provide a framework that support and protect the organs.

57. Connective tissues are separated by an _____ consisting of microscopic _____ scattered throughout a _____ secreted by the cells.

58. _____ fibers provide great strength to body structures, whereas fine branched _____ fibers support tissues and organs.

59. Tiny sacs in the lungs contain _____ fibers that stretch and recoil when air is inhaled and exhaled.

60. _____, found in connective tissue, are large cells that phagocytize cellular debris and bacteria.

Match the term on the left to the correct selection on the right. (Section V)

61. _____ adipose

62. _____ cartilage

63. _____ bone

64. _____ muscle

65. _____ skeletal

66. _____ cardiac

67. _____ smooth

68. _____ nervous

69. _____ sensory

70. _____ motor

A. consists of matrix containing osteocytes and osteons

B. muscle found in walls of the digestive tract; fibers are not striated

C. neurons that receive information from sensory receptors and transmit information to the brain and spinal cord

D. stores and releases fat as the body needs energy; provides insulation

E. neurons that transmit information from the brain and spinal cord to muscles and glands

F. tissue that receives and transmits messages; consists of neurons and glial cells

G. tissue found in vertebral disks and at the ends of bones

H. muscle found in the walls of the heart; striated muscle fibers characterized by intercalated disks

I. tissue composed of cells specialized to contract

J. muscles that are attached to bone; striated muscle fibers

Unscramble the names of the different membranes and match them to their definition. (Section VI)

71. ecrlaisv   lines body cavities that are open to the outside of the body

72. lvaiyons   lines body cavities that do not open to the outside of the body

73. rsseuo   portion of membrane attached to the wall of a cavity

74. umscuo   part of membranes that cover organs inside of a cavity

75. atplriea   connective tissue membrane that lines the joint cavities

Label the structures of the cell (Section I) and the phases of mitosis (Section IV).

76. Label the parts of the cell in Figure 2-1.

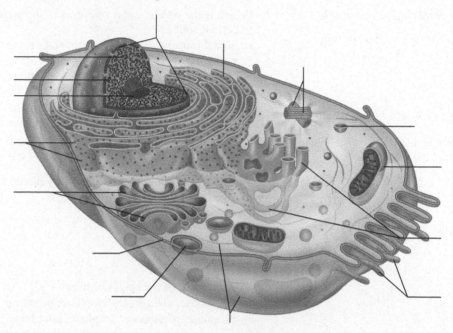

Figure 2-1

77. Label and describe each phase of mitosis in Figure 2-2.

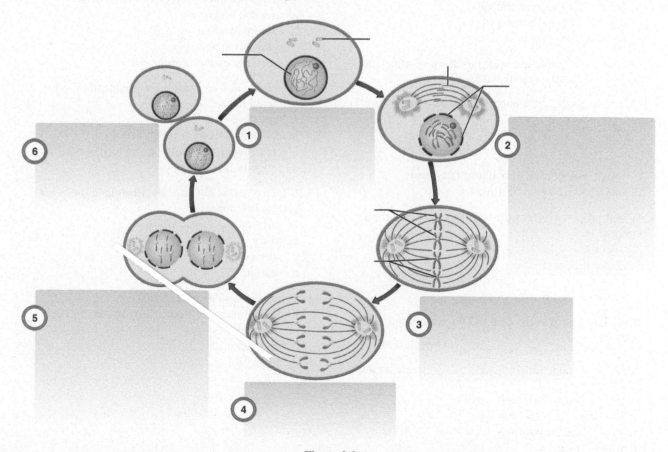

Figure 2-2

Select the correct answer.

1. Researchers use the greater resolving power of a(n)

   _____ to discern the fine details of thin cross-sections of cells.
   a. light microscope
   b. scanning electron microscope
   c. magnifying lens
   d. transmission electron microscope

2. Which of the following is not a cell?
   a. ovum
   b. lymphocyte
   c. ribosome
   d. sperm

3. Which organelle would not be found in the cytoplasm of a cell?
   a. nucleolus
   b. mitochondria
   c. endoplasmic reticulum
   d. ribosome

4. Which is not a function of smooth endoplasmic reticulum?
   a. synthesize steroids
   b. break down toxic chemicals
   c. ingest invading bacteria
   d. produce fatty acids

5. Cellular respiration, the breaking down of molecules and releasing their energy, takes place in

   _____; the energy released may be stored

   in _____.
   a. mitochondria; ATP
   b. Golgi complex; ATP
   c. rough endoplasmic reticulum; fatty acids
   d. mitochondria; phospholipids

6. Which process requires the cell to expend metabolic energy?
   a. diffusion
   b. active transport
   c. osmosis
   d. filtration

7. For active transport to occur, ATP provides the

   energy to pump _____ out of the cell,

   while at the same time, _____ are moved into the cell.
   a. potassium ions; sodium ions
   b. sodium ions; potassium ions
   c. free radicals; ribosomes
   d. water; gases

8. Which is the correct order of events in the process of cell signaling?
   a. signal transduction; signal sent; response; reception
   b. signal sent; signal transduction; reception; response
   c. signal sent; reception; signal transduction; response
   d. reception; signal transduction; signal sent; response

9. What must be duplicated before a cell can undergo mitosis?
   a. enzymes
   b. cell membrane
   c. chromosomes
   d. mitochondria

10. The sequence of the stages of mitosis is
    a. interphase, metaphase, telophase, prophase
    b. prophase, metaphase, anaphase, telophase
    c. metaphase, anaphase, interphase, telophase
    d. prophase, anaphase, metaphase, telophase

11. Which is not a function of epithelial cells?
    a. transmit messages
    b. excrete materials
    c. transport mucus
    d. receive sensory information

12. Which is not true concerning pseudostratified epithelial tissue?
    a. may have cilia
    b. contains cells of different heights
    c. cells may not extend to exposed tissue surface
    d. found in layers

13. Which gland is not an endocrine gland (does not secrete hormones)?
    a. salivary
    b. ovary
    c. adrenal
    d. thyroid

14. Intercellular substance consists of
    a. living materials produced by tissue
    b. microtubules
    c. secreted matrix
    d. collagen

Chapter **2** **Cells and Tissues**

15. Fibroblasts and macrophages are common in
    a. nervous tissue
    b. connective tissue
    c. muscle tissue
    d. adipose tissue

16. Which type of muscle fiber is striated and contains intercalated disks?
    a. cardiac
    b. smooth
    c. connective
    d. skeletal

17. A neuron consists of
    a. cell body, dendrites, and lacunae
    b. axon, dendrites, and intercalated disk
    c. dendrites, lacunae, and axon
    d. cell body, axon, and dendrites

18. Which is not true concerning a mucous membrane?
    a. does not open to the outside of the body
    b. lines the digestive tract
    c. secretes mucus
    d. lines body cavities that open to the outside of the body

PART 3: ACCEPT THE CHALLENGE

1. Describe a condition in which excess adipose tissue could be harmful.

2. How could mitosis be affected if cells did not enter interphase, but immediately began the next mitotic cycle?

3. Is the release of hormones directly into tissue fluid an advantage? Explain.

Find and circle the following words from Chapter 2. Words may be found from top to bottom, bottom to top, right to left, left to right, and diagonally.

```
S L B Q T O T I L D I S I S O T I M N K T A R Y G W D P R K
X H G A J F D T X E R W P K K K V V O D I A Z L R X R P C G
G O F O U F Z Z S S L V Y C R Q O E A L B Q R M Q Q Y J N O
Y Q W H E B V E B A J I W A W R Z A L R Q P R C Q I T V A J
B K Y R I Q N G P H P N X R M Y C J Y A C Z A N Q Q C K E V
S N Z U W E D E E P V T U P N N U C L E A R E N V E L O P E
K G K D G V I N H A E E J H I K H W B Z A L S V F F X Z E A
G B W V O I D O B N N R Y C H R O M O S O M E S J W E U D N
F M J I M J V M G A H P A N G B T I H U G E L P I M E G X B
L U G Y Z T J E H H U H C P S D E E J F Y T P U A V F P F T
T M T W Z N D Z P M Y A K V H I E X W I D C T K A N M Z V N
X C E C Y Z Q R L W P S G B O S S Z Y N I F M E P P S G K Z
J X B G M A K Q A C I E S T B Q K O H R B B S B Q A A G C G
X T O I V X F Y S F U Y Q M A A E V I E U G L N H P L F K F
F R K L O F A W M A Z E A F Y Y X K B E X R Y B L E P P Z N
E G Y S L M R X A Z H D Z E F B K G G K M G D W H C O N G G
B M X U C C D I M A O W T M W A R X G W Y Q E G A L T L X U
Q M A E W N P T E P R W A T M W M Y U M R S T O S L Y U B O
F M N L A C Z C M A P M I T O C H O N D R I A R T G C I R G
B E F C P E Z E B W T Z M O K G P A O B N O G P S G E K C K
U T T U Y X A N R C Z P R O P H A S E T O A V S M J D U Y D
I D B N T Y H I A R Q M B S Y X L T V L R T L N V E E P Q X
B N B C X B H G N C A E K I V A W Y U V G W F Q T L Q K E F
H A J U Z G X A E K V B V B D S H P C F A R Z D L O W B T M
V J Y Z R F I N E Q L G C A H U J N O S N E Q X W I R B J M
C C C X O C Z H I J U O A F C E N C Y Y E P O R U R F O S Y
R D O W I S T W U S F C E Z R U H O K W L Q J X I T X O E E
E W F W B T U J L N H H I M M M O F S V L T C T J N N Q T N
E X M E T A P H A S E T L V Y J X L D I E E S Q O E C C A O
Q F I N A N H L C X F P E E J P A J E Z S D B H H C V X X Y
```

anaphase

centriole

chromosomes

cytoplasm

DNA

genes

genome

interphase

meiosis

metaphase

mitochondria

mitosis

nuclear envelope

nucleus

organelles

plasma membrane

prophase

vacuole

Chapter **2** **Cells and Tissues**

3 | The Integumentary System

CHAPTER GUIDE

I.   The integumentary system protects the body
II. The skin consists of the epidermis and dermis
   A. The epidermis continuously replaces itself
   B. The dermis provides strength and elasticity
   C. The subcutaneous layer attaches the skin to underlying tissues

III. The skin has specialized accessory structures
   A. The hair shaft consists of dead cells
   B. Sebaceous glands lubricate the hair and skin
   C. Sweat glands help maintain body temperature
   D. Nails protect the ends of the fingers and toes
IV. Melanin helps determine skin color

LEARNING OBJECTIVES

1. List six functions of the integumentary system and explain how each is important for maintaining homeostasis.
2. Compare the structure and functions of the epidermis with that of the dermis.
3. Relate the structure of the subcutaneous layer with its functions.
4. Describe the structure of a hair.
5. Describe the functions of sebaceous glands.
6. Connect the functions of sweat glands with homeostasis of the body.
7. Relate the structure of nails to their function.
8. Describe two functions of melanin.

PART 1: LEARN THE TERMS

Match the following terms to the correct definitions by writing the corresponding letter in the space provided. (Sections I and II)

A. **dermal papillae**   B. **dermis**   C. **epidermis**   D. **integumentary**
E. **keratin**   F. **stratum basale** G. **stratum corneum** H. **superficial fascia**

1. _____ outer sublayer of the epidermis

2. _____ fingerlike extensions that project into the epidermis

3. _____ subcutaneous layer beneath the dermis

4. _____ thick layer of skin beneath the epidermis

5. _____ tough waterproofing protein made by epidermal cells

6. _____ outer layer of skin consisting of stratified squamous epithelial tissue

7. _____ deepest sublayer of the epidermis

8. _____ organ system made up of skin, hair, nails, and glands

Fill in the blank with the correct answer for each statement. (Section III)

9. The _____ is the part of the hair above the skin surface.

10. The _____ of the hair is below the skin surface, and along with associated epithelial and connective tissue coverings, makes up the _____.

11. _____ are generally attached to hair follicles by tiny ducts.

12. _____ is an oily substance secreted by sebaceous glands, which lubricates the hair and skin.

13. When sebum in a duct becomes infected by bacteria, it forms a _____.

14. Sebaceous glands become more active during puberty and can cause _____.

15. _____ in the dermis and subcutaneous tissue help the skin maintain body temperature.

16. Sweat glands excrete excess _____, _____, and small amounts of nitrogen wastes.

Unscramble the parts of the nail and match them to their definition. (Section III)

17. ebd alin   A. actively growing part of the nail

18. llnauu   B. closely compressed protein

19. yobd ainl   C. layer of epithelium below the nail

20. rtusamt laseba   D. white crescent at the base of a nail

21. ntkriea   E. visible part of the nail

Fill in the blanks to complete each sequential step of the cell signaling process, and then unscramble the circled letters to correctly complete the final sentence. (Section IV)

22. _ _ ◯ _ _ ◯ _ _, a yellow pigment found in carrots, helps to determine skin color.

23. Pigment cells, or _ _ _ _ ◯ _ _ _ _ ◯, are scattered through the lowest layer of the epidermis and produce melanin.

24. Excessive exposure to ◯ _ _ _ _ _ _ _ _ _ radiation from the sun over many years can cause

_ _ _ _ ◯ _ _ _ _.

25. _ ◯ _ _ _ _ _ gives color to the skin and hair; it is a protective screen against the harmful ultraviolet rays of the sun.

26. An inherited condition in which cells do not produce melanin is called _ _ _ _ ◯ _ ◯ _.

27. Use _ _ _ _ _ _ _ _ _ to reduce the risk of skin cancer and excessive wrinkling.

28. Label the parts of the skin in Figure 3-1.

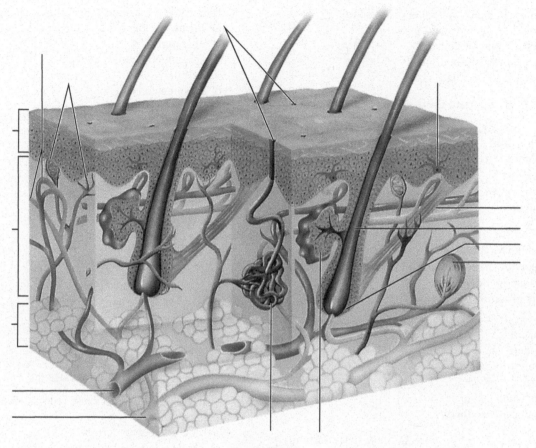

Figure 3-1

29. Label the parts of the nail in Figure 3-2.

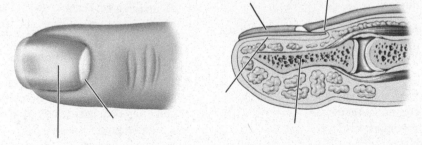

Figure 3-2

Select the correct answer.

1. The integumentary system is made up of
   a. skin, bone, glands, and nerves
   b. nerves, skin, and glands
   c. skin, hair, nails, and glands
   d. skin, hair, bone, and nails

2. The skin is important for maintaining

   _____, the body's balanced internal
   environment.
   a. mitosis
   b. homeostasis
   c. metabolism
   d. anabolism

3. Which of the following is not a function of the skin?
   a. making vitamin D
   b. receiving and communicating information
   c. producing bone tissue
   d. part of temperature regulating system

4. The _____ consists of several sublayers

   of squamous _____ tissue.
   a. epidermis; epithelial
   b. dermis; collagen
   c. epidermis; adipose
   d. epidermis; connective

5. The _____ contains cells that constantly

   divide by _____, producing millions of
   new cells each day.
   a. stratum basale; osmosis
   b. stratum corneum; mitosis
   c. subcutaneous layer; meiosis
   d. stratum basale; mitosis

6. New epidermal cells are pushed upward from the

   _____ and die as they move through the

   _____.
   a. subcutaneous layer; stratum basale
   b. stratum basale; stratum corneum
   c. stratum basale; subcutaneous layer
   d. stratum corneum; stratum basale

7. The _____ is directly below the
   epidermis and is composed mainly of

   _____ fibers.
   a. subcutaneous layer; collagen
   b. dermis; nerve
   c. dermis; collagen
   d. stratum corneum; muscle

8. Blood vessels, nerves, hair follicles, and glands are
   all located in the _____.
   a. epidermis
   b. stratum corneum
   c. dermis
   d. subcutaneous layer

9. The _____ project into the epidermal
   tissue and provide oxygen and nutrients to
   epidermal cells through networks of

   _____
   a. hair follicles; fibers
   b. nerve ends; receptors
   c. hair follicles; capillaries
   d. dermal papillae; capillaries

10. The _____ layer consists of loose

    connective tissue and _____ tissue.
    a. subcutaneous; adipose
    b. subcutaneous; dense connective
    c. dermal; adipose
    d. epidermal; dense connective

11. _____ burns damage the

    _____ and cause redness, swelling, and
    pain.
    a. first-degree; epidermis
    b. second-degree; subcutaneous layer
    c. first-degree; dermis
    d. third-degree; epidermis

12. _____ burns damage the epidermis and

    dermis; they cause _____ to form.
    a. first-degree; scars
    b. second-degree; blisters
    c. second-degree; pimples
    d. first-degree; blisters

13. _____ burns, which require immediate
    emergency medical attention, damage all skin layers
    and often damage underlying tissue.
    a. first-degree
    b. second-degree
    c. third-degree
    d. first- and second-degree

14. Epidermal cells from the stratum basale push down into the _____ where they multiply and develop into _____ and

    _____.
    a. dermis; capillaries; nerves
    b. stratum corneum; hair follicles; glands
    c. subcutaneous layer; nerves; glands
    d. dermis; hair follicles; glands

15. Hair is found on most skin surfaces except
    a. soles of feet, palms, and genitals
    b. soles of feet, palms, and lips
    c. nose, palms, and lips
    d. nose, genitals, and lips

16. A hair follicle is made up of the
    a. shaft and root
    b. root with epithelial and connective tissue coverings
    c. shaft, root with epithelial and connective tissue coverings, and surrounding tissue
    d. root with epithelial and connective tissue coverings, and surrounding tissue

17. Sebaceous glands are most numerous on the

    _____ and _____.
    a. face; scalp
    b. face; underarms
    c. scalp; underarms
    d. face; palms

18. Sebaceous glands are directed by _____

    to secrete more _____ during puberty.
    a. nerves; sebum
    b. nerves; keratin
    c. hormones; sebum
    d. hormones; acne

19. The body sweats profusely under strenuous exercise

    requiring _____ and salts to be quickly

    replaced to help maintain _____.
    a. water; respiration
    b. food; weight
    c. water; homeostasis
    d. food; respiration

20. The _____ is rich in _____, which gives the nail a pink color.
    a. nail body; nutrients
    b. nail bed; nutrients
    c. nail bed; capillaries
    d. nail bed; melanin

21. The actively growing area of the nail is in

    _____ below the _____ at the base of the nail.
    a. stratum basale; lunula
    b. stratum corneum; stratum basale
    c. stratum basale; bone
    d. stratum corneum; knuckle

22. People with more _____ in their skin

    have _____ skin.
    a. melanin; dryer
    b. carotene; dryer
    c. melanin; lighter
    d. melanin; darker

23. When skin is exposed to excessive ultraviolet radiation, melanin
    a. decreases
    b. increases
    c. disappears
    d. none of the above

24. The incidence of _____ is increasing more rapidly than any other type of cancer due to exposure to the sun.
    a. basal cell carcinoma
    b. squamous cell carcinoma
    c. malignant melanoma
    d. leukemia

1. Why do medical caregivers record information about your skin during an exam? What type of specialist might you be referred to if you have a skin disease?

2. What are the most serious concerns for a patient being treated for burns that have destroyed large areas of skin? What treatment might be recommended?

3. What happens when excessive skin cells on the scalp are sloughed off and mix with sebum from the hair?

THE PUZZLE

Answer the questions to complete the crossword puzzle.

Skin Game

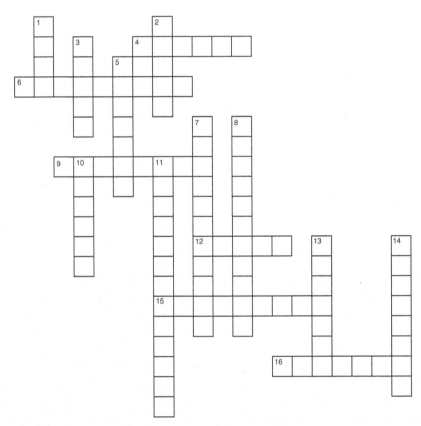

Across

4. thick layer of skin beneath the epidermis
6. gland that is generally attached to hair follicle
9. condition in which a person is born unable to produce melanin
12. degree number of burn that is most serious
15. outer layer of skin consisting of stratified squamous epithelial tissue
16. tough waterproofing protein made by epidermal cells

Down

1. skin scourge of teenagers
2. secreted by sebaceous glands
3. part of hair that is seen above the epidermis
5. dark pigment that colors and protects skin
7. skin helps the body maintain this normal state
8. this radiation from sun causes cancer
10. white crescent at the base of the nail
11. organ system that protects outside of body
13. sore produced by second-degree burn
14. yellow pigment in skin

Chapter **3** **The Integumentary System**

4 The Skeletal System

LEARNING OBJECTIVES

1. List five functions of the skeletal system.
2. Describe the gross and microscopic structure of a typical bone.
3. Contrast endochondral with intramembranous bone development.
4. Describe the functions of osteoblasts and osteoclasts in bone production and remodeling.
5. Distinguish between the axial skeleton and the appendicular skeleton.
6. Identify the bones of the axial skeleton. (Locate each bone on a diagram or skeleton.)
7. Describe and give the function of each of the cranial and facial bones.
8. Describe the regions of the vertebral column, and identify the bones and functions of the vertebral column and thoracic cage.
9. Describe and give the function of each of the bones of the appendicular skeleton. (Locate each on a diagram or skeleton.)
10. Describe and give the function of each bone of the pectoral girdle, upper extremity, pelvic girdle, and lower extremity. (Locate each bone on a diagram or skeleton.)
11. Compare the main types of joints.
12. Describe the structure and functions of a diarthrosis.
13. Describe each type of body movement.

PART 1: LEARN THE TERMS

Fill in the blank with the correct answer for each statement. (Section I)

1. The skeletal system provides _____ to the body by serving as a bony framework for the other tissues and organs.

2. The strong bones of the skeletal system _____ delicate vital organs.

3. Bones serve as _____ that transmit muscular forces.

4. _____ are bands of connective tissue that attach muscles to bones.

5. Parts of the body move when a _____ contracts, pulling the attached _____.

6. _____ are bands of connective tissue that hold bones together at the _____.

7. Blood cells are produced by the _____ in some bones.

8. Bones store and release minerals, including _____ and _____.

Match the following terms to the correct definitions by writing the corresponding letter in the space provided. (Section II)

A. articular cartilage	**B. bone marrow**	**C. compact**	**D. diaphysis**	**E. endosteum**
F. epiphyses	**G. haversian canals**	**H. lacunae**	**I. metaphysis**	**J. osteocytes**
K. osteons	**L. periosteum**	**M. red**	**N. spongy**	**O. yellow**

9. _____ thin layer of cells that line the yellow marrow cavity

10. _____ outer layer of a joint surface (consists of a thin layer of hyaline cartilage)

11. _____ bone found within the epiphyses; makes up the inner part of the wall of the diaphysis

12. _____ layer of connective tissue covering bones containing cells that produce bone

13. _____ fills the spaces within spongy bone

14. _____ mature bone cells located within each osteon

15. _____ very dense, hard bone found near bone surfaces where strength is important

16. _____ main shaft of a long bone

17. _____ marrow that contains numerous fat storage cells

18. _____ bone growth center in children found between the epiphysis and diaphysis

19. _____ interlocking, spindle-shaped units that make up compact bone

20. _____ small cavities arranged in concentric circles around central haversian canals

21. _____ expanded end of a bone

22. _____ bone marrow in which blood cells are manufactured

23. _____ blood vessels that nourish bone cells pass through these

24. Label the parts of the bone in Figure 4-1.

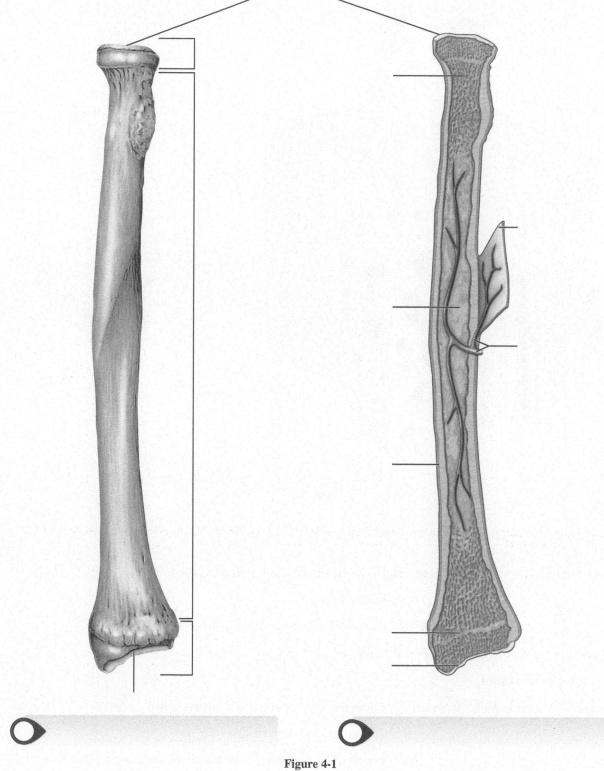

Figure 4-1

25. Label the parts of the bone in Figure 4-2.

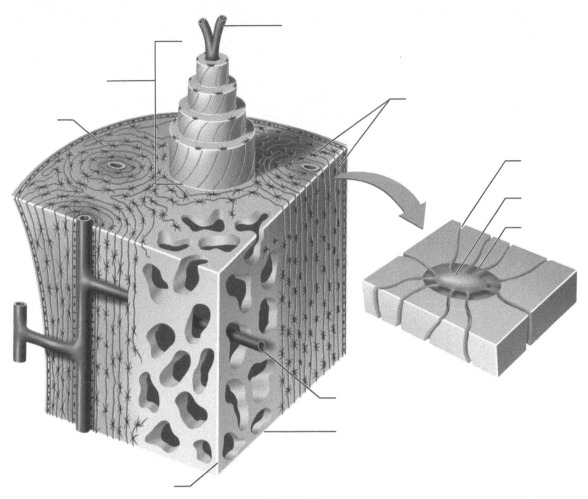

Figure 4-2

Fill in the blanks to complete each sentence, and then unscramble the circled letters to correctly complete the final sentence. (Section III)

26. Long bones develop from a cartilage template in the fetus through a process called

_ _ _ _ _ _ _ _ _ _ _ ◯ _ bone development.

27. _ _ _ ◯ _ _ _ _ _ _ _ _ are cells that produce bone by secreting the protein collagen.

28. Osteoclasts are very large cells that break down, or ◯ _ _ _ _ _ _, bone.

29. Bone formation is called _ _ _ _ _ ◯ _ _ _ _ _ _ _.

30. Some bones develop from a non-cartilage connective tissue scaffold in a process called

_ _ _ _ _ _ _ _ _ _ _ _ _ _ _ ◯ _ bone development.

31. _ _ _ _ _ _ _ _ ◯ _ _ _ _ _ may develop when bone tissue is broken down more quickly than it is produced.

32. _ _ _ _ _ ◯ _ _ _ _ _ resorb bone by secreting enzymes that digest collagen and hydrogen ions that dissolve crystals.

33. When osteoblasts become embedded in the bone matrix, they are called _ _ _ _ _ _ _ ◯ _ _.

34. A _ _ _ _ _ _ _ _ _ is a crack or break in a bone.

Match the term on the left to the correct selection on the right. (Section IV and V)

35. _____ sagittal suture

36. _____ skull

37. _____ axial skeleton

38. _____ coronal suture

39. _____ sinuses

40. _____ appendicular skeleton

41. _____ fontanelles

42. _____ cranium

43. _____ sutures

44. _____ lambdoid suture

A. bones of the upper and lower extremities and bones that attach extremities to the axial skeleton

B. air-filled spaces lined with mucous membranes

C. joint between the two parietal bones in the midline

D. set of eight bones that enclose the brain

E. joint between the parietal bones and occipital bone (close space between occipital and bone)

F. bones that form the central axis of the body

G. joins the parietal bones to the frontal bone

H. the bony framework of the head

I. joints in a baby's skull where ossification is not yet complete

J. immoveable joints that join the bones of the skull

45. Label the parts of the skull in Figure 4-3.

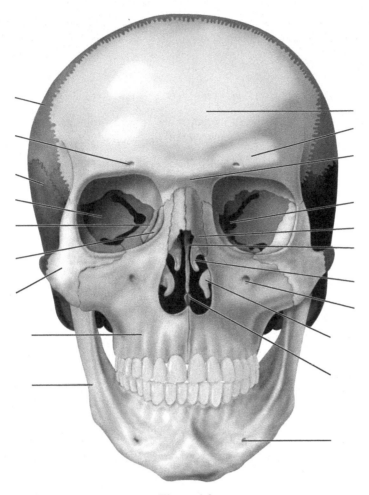

Figure 4-3

46. Label the parts of the skull in Figure 4-4.

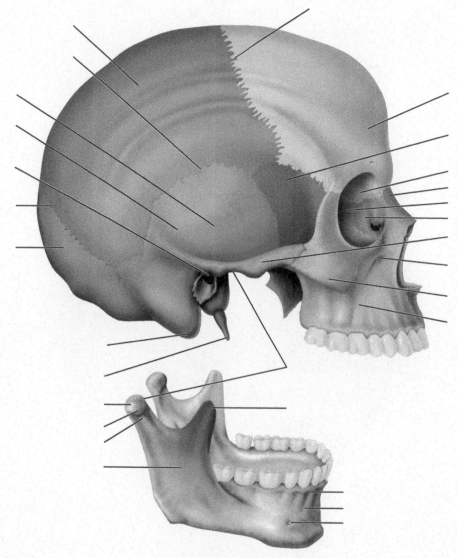

Figure 4-4

47. Label the parts of the skull in Figure 4-5.

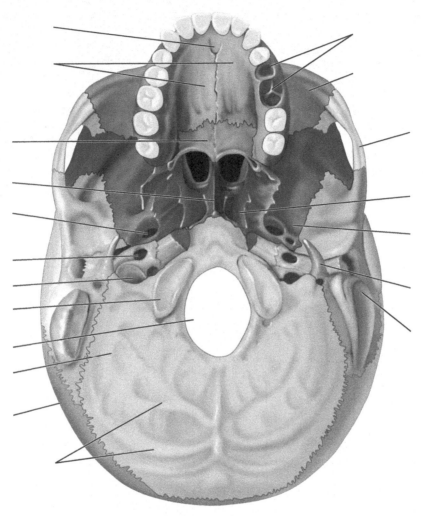

Figure 4-5

Fill in the blank with the correct answer for each statement. (Section V)

48. The _____ column supports the body and protects the spinal cord.

49. The two fused bones at the base of the vertebral column are the _____ and the _____.

50. The neck, or _____ region, of the vertebral column consists of _____ vertebrae.

51. The _____, or chest region, of the vertebral column has 12 vertebrae.

52. The _____, or back region, of the vertebral column contains five vertebrae.

53. The pelvic, or _____ region, is a single bone (sacrum) composed of _____ fused vertebrae; the _____ area is made up of three to five fused vertebrae.

54. The _____, composed of cartilage, are tiny pads that act as shock absorbers.

55. A vertebra consists of an anterior region called the _____ and a posterior, curved area called the _____.

56. Lateral regions of the posterior part of a vertebra are the _____.

57. The _____ are lateral projections from the centrum, which have articular surfaces for connecting with other vertebrae and ribs.

58. The _____, made up of adjacent _____, encases the spinal cord.

59. The _____, or rib cage, provides support for the bones of the pectoral girdle and upper extremities and is important in breathing.

60. The _____, or breast bone, thoracic vertebrae, and _____ pairs of ribs form the thoracic cage.

61. Label the parts of the vertebral column and vertebrae in Figure 4-6.

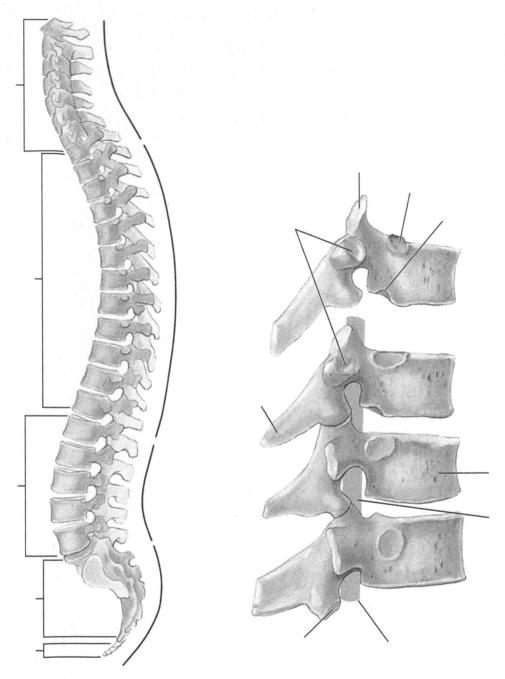

Figure 4-6

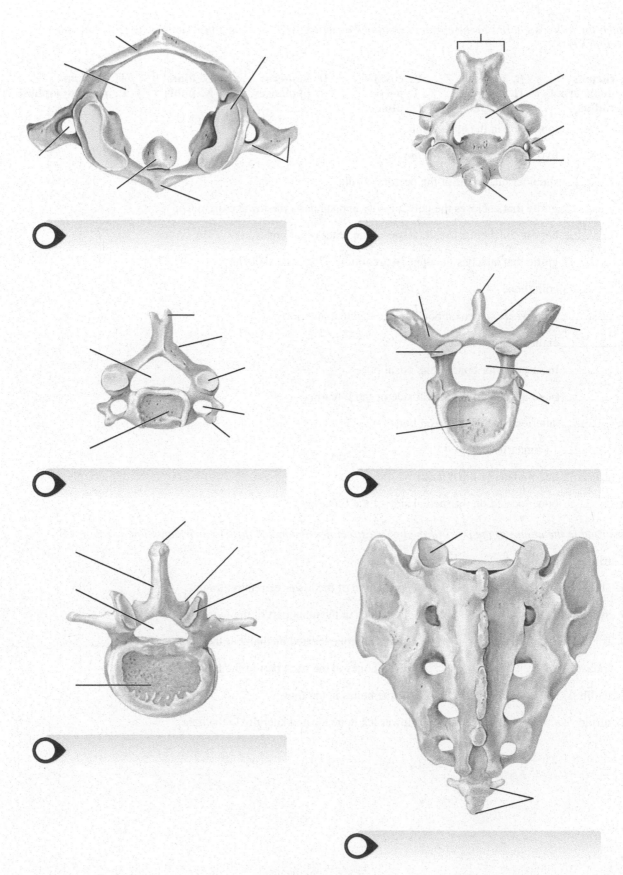

Figure 4-6—cont'd

Match the following terms to the correct definitions by writing the corresponding letter in the space provided. (Section VI)

A. carpals	**B. clavicle**	**C. coxal**	**D. humerus**	**E. ilium**	**F. ischium**
G. metacarpals	**H. pectoral**	**I. pelvic**	**J. phalanges**	**K. pubis**	**L. pubic symphysis**
M. radius	**N. scapula**	**O. ulna**			

62. _____ long bone in the upper limb

63. _____ five bones in the palm of the hand

64. _____ shoulder blade half of the pectoral girdle

65. _____ girdle that encloses the pelvic cavity and supports the lower extremities

66. _____ largest coxal bone found on top of the other coxal bones

67. _____ girdle that attaches the upper extremities to the axial skeleton

68. _____ collarbone

69. _____ joint where the coxal bones come together anteriorly

70. _____ eight small wrist bones

71. _____ most posterior bone of the coxal bone

72. _____ bone located on the lateral side of the forearm

73. _____ anterior bone of the coxal bone

74. _____ 14 finger bones

75. _____ innominate, or hip bones

76. _____ bone located on the medial side of the forearm

Unscramble the names of the parts of the lower extremities and match them to their definition. (Section VI)

77. trlmtaeassa   kneecap

78. abiti   upper limb of the lower extremity; thigh

79. apsghlnea   five bones in the main part of the foot

80. lstrsaa   lower leg bone located medially to the fibula

81. lptlaae   seven bones in the back part of the foot and heel

82. uafbli   14 toe bones in the foot

83. ufrme   lower leg bone located laterally to the tibia

84. Label the parts of the hand in Figure 4-7.

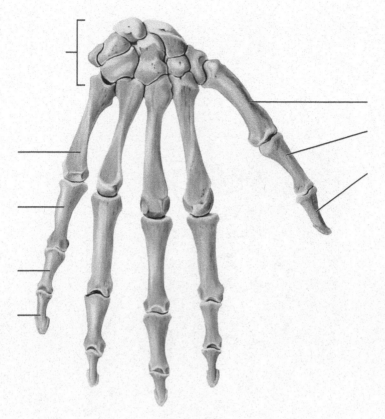

Figure 4-7

85. Label the parts of the foot in Figure 4-8.

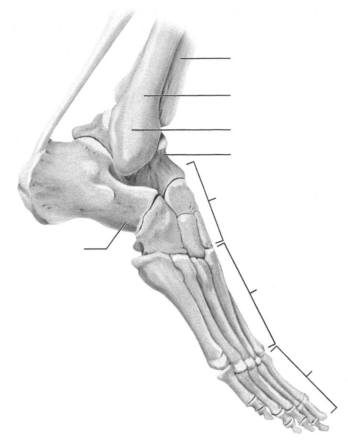

Figure 4-8

Fill in the blank with the correct answer for each statement. (Section VII)

86. A joint, or _____, is a point of contact between two bones.

87. _____ permit slight movement and help absorb shock; the bones are joined by cartilage.

88. Joints that do not permit movement, such as the sutures that join skull bones are called _____.

89. Diarthroses, or _____ joints, are freely movable joints, but their _____ varies.

90. A diarthrodial joint is surrounded by a connective tissue capsule, the _____, made of tough, fibrous connective tissue.

91. The joint capsule is reinforced with bands of fibrous connective tissue, called _____, that connect the bones and also limit movement at the joint.

92. A membrane in the joint capsule secrets a lubricant called _____, which reduces _____ during movement and absorbs shock.

93. Fluid-filled sacs called _____, located between bone and tendons, and between bone and some other tissues, cushion the movement of bone over other tissues.

94. Movement of a bone, or limb, away from the midline of the body is called _____; movement of a bone, or limb, toward the midline is called _____.

95. Label the parts of the knee joint in Figure 4-9.

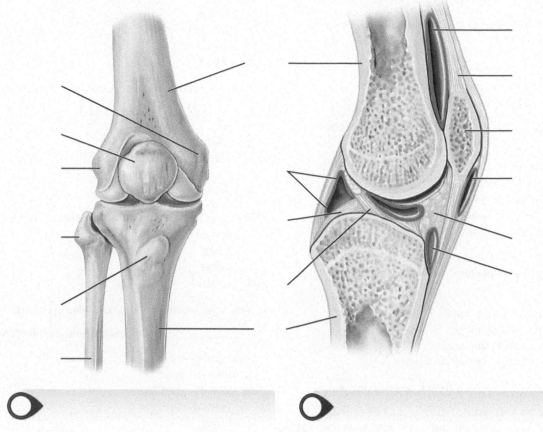

Figure 4-9

PART 2: ASSESS YOUR UNDERSTANDING

Select the correct answer.

1. Which of the following is *not* a function of the skeleton?
   a. support
   b. protect
   c. circulate blood
   d. store minerals

2. The growth centers of bones are the

   _____.

   a. metaphyses
   b. epiphyses
   c. endosteum
   d. diaphysis

3. Blood cells are manufactured in the _____
   a. yellow marrow
   b. compact bone
   c. osteocytes
   d. red marrow

4. In adults blood cells are produced by the

   _____, _____, and

   _____.

   a. vertebrae; sternum; pelvis
   b. sternum; ribs; fibula
   c. clavicle; pelvis; humerus
   d. fibula; vertebrae; ribs

5. The skeleton of a fetus consists mainly of

_____ with long bones developing from

a template in a process called _____
bone development.
   a. bone; fetal
   b. cartilage; endochondral
   c. cartilage; intramembranous
   d. bone; ossification

6. _____ are the cells that produce bone by

secreting _____ to produce strong,
elastic bone fibers.
   a. Osteoclasts; calcium
   b. Osteoblasts; enzymes
   c. Osteoblasts; collagen
   d. Osteoclasts; enzymes

7. Osteocytes are found in _____, which
are arranged in concentric circles around central

_____.
   a. osteons; haversian canals
   b. spongy bone; cartilage
   c. lacuna; haversian canals
   d. yellow marrow; haversian canals

8. _____ resorb (break down) bone and

work side by side with _____ to shape
bones and to form the precise grain needed in the
finished bone.
   a. osteoclasts; osteoblasts
   b. osteoblasts; osteons
   c. osteoclasts; osteons
   d. osteoblasts; osteoclasts

9. The axial skeleton consists of the _____

_____, _____, and sternum.
   a. skull; clavicle; ribs
   b. skull; vertebral column; ribs
   c. scapula; clavicle; vertebral column
   d. skull; pelvis; scapula

10. The adult skull consists of _____ bones
and six very small bones in the middle ears called

the _____.
   a. 18; alveolar process
   b. 22; auditory ossicles
   c. 22; alveolar process
   d. 14; auditory ossicles

11. The two parietal bones are joined in the midline by

the _____ suture.
   a. coronal
   b. lambdoid
   c. parietal
   d. sagittal

12. The paranasal sinuses are located in the frontal,

_____, sphenoid, and _____
bones.
   a. maxillary; ethmoid
   b. occipital; ethmoid
   c. maxillary; parietal
   d. parietal; ethmoid

13. Which is not a region of the vertebral column?
   a. cervical
   b. cranial
   c. lumbar
   d. sacral

14. Vertebrae articulate with each other by means of

_____ joints and by means of intervertebral

disks composed of _____.
   a. synovial; bone
   b. inflexible; cartilage
   c. synovial; cartilage
   d. sliding; bone

15. The thoracic cage contains _____ pairs
of ribs, which protect the internal organs of the

_____.
   a. 12; thoracic cavity
   b. 24; pelvic cavity
   c. 24; thoracic cavity
   d. 12; pelvic cavity

Mark each statement true or false; correct the false statements to make them true.

16. _____ The pectoral girdle attaches the upper limbs to the axial skeleton.

17. _____ The pectoral girdle articulates with the sternum but not with the vertebral column.

18. _____ A "typical" vertebra consists of two main parts, the centrum and neural arch.

19. _____ The coxal bones, together with the scapula and coccyx, form the pelvic girdle.

20. _____ Each coxal bone is formed from the fusion of three bones (ilium, ischium, and pubis) during development.

21. _____ The female pelvis is broader and more shallow than the male pelvis and has a lesser angle between the pubic bones to accommodate childbirth.

22. _____ Joints hold bones together and can be classified in three main groups based on the degree of movement they permit.

23. _____ Most of the body's joints are diarthroses, or synovial joints, and are referred to as immovable joints.

24. _____ The joint capsule is typically reinforced with tendons that connect the bones and also limit movement at the joint.

25. _____ Bursae are located between bone and tendons, and between bone and some other tissues; they cushion the movement of bone over other tissues.

26. Label the parts of the skeleton in Figure 4-10.

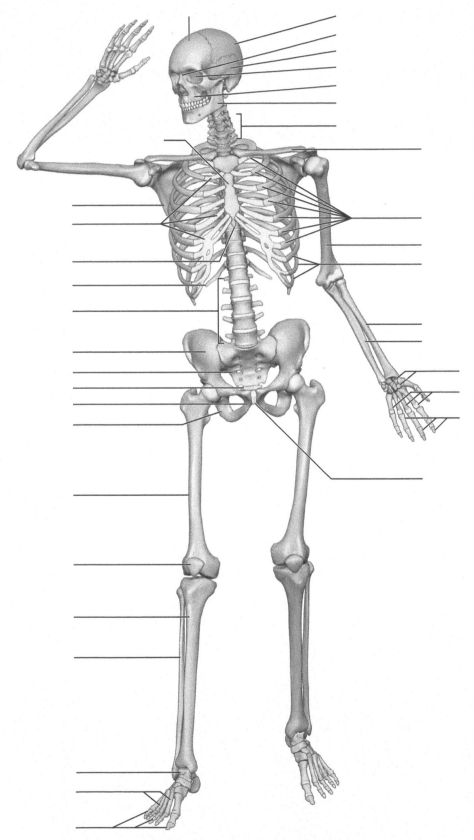

Figure 4-10

PART 3: ACCEPT THE CHALLENGE

1. How might women reduce the risks and effects of osteoporosis as they age?

2. How is the structure of the foot different from that of the hand? Why?

3. Can you think of a situation where a strong thoracic cage could be a disadvantage?

THE PUZZLE

Find and circle the following words from Chapter 4. Words may be found from top to bottom, bottom to top, right to left, left to right, and diagonally.

```
E C Y U E R W G S C M E T W S F X Z P M T Q H A Q I Z Q Y H
R O Z U H W V C V W S J E U I S R N T N W R H R I S E M B Q
D S D J X U Q F C C H F L B S K O P T O J W S P W D W L U S
V I V F M O L U Q I F T K C Y K X P R E B X C U W U A O T A
Z T U N X R X N H P V F O V H J D V S T B B R P R I K W R S
M B R G V B R T A I H M O J P L I J B S C P O U X E K H G L
N A Y O Z I A J G N Y O I O A V G V N O W U R A Y H M P K G
J A H U E H L L N A F L O U I I U U S P V V O A Y N P U C U
S C I C D G U Q J U R Y I U D J P N R B Z E P K Q F P Z H Q
T O E S B Y C T S S I W Q B I W Q L V C J H C X P F X G I R
E K C B X I I R Q G S A C B G U D G G T N E M A G I L J B B
R X L K D F D J K F O S U N B N H O Y B S Y Q U W W V Q P U
N I E V X C N G B D E A X J A Z J Y P Q P C F T V E Z W V H
U T F F K K E L O S B D Y K Z H C V M K Z S S V O M N G A Z
M U I H G L P X A A Y R R T Y N G R M F F V K C Q L Q O I U
F S H G P V P L Z Y Q L U E J A C P I R Q K V S P Q N R B N
G T N X C E A Y G N Z S O W E J S E I T I M E R T X E D O F
A Y W Q I C Y T Y A P E L V I S U B Y Q E R G H D Z B W H H
A Q G C X P O L R G R U M E F Z F F T A E X V Q F U G I R L
W Z H J W R Z C O V Y X P T O S C C R A N I U M D S G W R Q
Y D M Q E Z X L C J R U P I N I I D Q U K G G Q F C R N C J
M M I M U G K C Q Y Z V E R T E B R A E O C G B S Z E Q P S
K L U K W G V S U T X B G Y V G E D S Z J T H F M Z O H J T
I T V G D Q J I L A D M L Z U B M W O A M L Y V Q N V P V H
H K F G E Z G Y D C V T K W X G A H N M E T A C A R P A L F
M G O I K R O V W X I I M W Q V P Q S W U B Z G Z S O D P Y
F B G H O O J L E B Z N X O O C A L D C E A T P Y U N W Q P
V C J E B W M I I Y I U O K B Z S G W Y O C O U J Z Z V H E
M P J G Z A M A Y O G F M I D V H Z S S W M U K A F M X H U
Z Z L D F Q A F A V V C H L V G A Y B Y V T J W T O A U X F
```

appendicular
axial
bone
coccyx
cranium
diaphysis
extremities
femur
humerus

ligament
metacarpal
osteon
pelvis
rib
sternum
tibia
ulna
vertebrae

5 | The Muscular System

I. A skeletal muscle is composed of hundreds of muscle fibers
II. Muscle fibers are specialized for contraction
   A. Muscle contraction occurs when actin and myosin filaments slide past each other
   B. Muscle contraction requires energy
   C. Muscle tone is a state of partial contraction
   D. Two types of contraction are isotonic and isometric
III. Muscles work antagonistically to one another
IV. We can study muscles in functional groups

LEARNING OBJECTIVES

1. Describe the structure of a skeletal muscle.
2. Relate the structure of a muscle fiber to its function.
3. List, in sequence, the events that take place during muscle contraction.
4. Compare the roles of glycogen, creatine phosphate, and ATP in providing energy for muscle contraction.
5. Define muscle tone and explain why it is important.
6. Compare isotonic and isometric contraction.
7. Explain how muscles work antagonistically to one another.
8. Locate and list the actions of the principal muscles as described in Table 5-1 in the textbook.

PART 1: LEARN THE TERMS

Match the term on the left to the correct selection on the right. (Section I)

1. _____ perimysium

2. _____ fascia

3. _____ epimysium

4. _____ fascicle

5. _____ endomysium

6. _____ skeletal muscle

7. _____ muscle fibers

8. _____ tendon

A. voluntary muscle attached to bone

B. cells that make up each skeletal muscle

C. bundle of muscle fibers

D. surrounds the muscle and merges with the tissue of the tendon

E. tough cords of connective tissue that anchor muscles to bones

F. connective tissue that covers individual muscle fibers

G. connective tissue that wraps a fascicle

H. connective tissue that covers a muscle

Match the following terms to the correct definitions by writing the corresponding letter in the space provided. (Section II)

A. actin
E. sarcomere
B. muscle filament
F. striation
C. myofibril
G. transverse tubules
D. myosin
H. Z line

9. _____ contractile protein that forms thick filaments

10. _____ inward extensions of the plasma membrane that surround myofibrils

11. _____ basic unit of muscle contraction made of actin and myosin filaments

12. _____ interwoven filament that joins sarcomeres at their ends

13. _____ pattern of transverse bands made up of overlapping muscle filaments

14. _____ protein threads that compose myofibrils

15. _____ contractile protein that forms thin filaments

16. _____ threadlike structure that runs lengthwise through the muscle fiber

Fill in the blank with the correct answer for each statement. (Section II)

17. Muscle _____ occurs when actin and myosin filaments slide past each other.

18. A muscle pulls on a _____ by contracting, or shortening, when its _____ contract.

19. A motor nerve is made up of motor _____ that transmit impulses to muscle fibers signaling them to

_____

20. Neurotransmitters send signals across _____, junctions between neurons or between a neuron and an

_____, a muscle or gland.

21. The neurotransmitter _____, a signaling molecule, is released into the _____ between the
motor neuron and the muscle fiber.

22. Acetylcholine diffuses across the synaptic cleft and combines with _____ on the surface of the muscle

fiber causing _____.

23. Depolarization may cause an electrical impulse, or _____, to be generated in the muscle fiber which

travels along the _____ and spreads through the T tubules.

24. Depolarization of the T tubules triggers release of stored _____ ions from the endoplasmic reticulum;

these ions bind to proteins on the _____, causing them to change shape and expose binding sites.

25. When binding sites are exposed, _____ is split and energy is released which energizes

_____

26. Energized myosin attaches to the _____ on the actin filament, forming a _____ that links
the myosin and actin filaments.

27. Release of inorganic phosphate from the _____ causes the cross bridges to flex pulling the actin

filament closer to the center of the _____ and shortening the muscle.

*Fill in the blanks to correctly complete each sentence, and then unscramble the circled letters to correctly complete the
final sentence. (Section II)*

28. Muscle fibers stockpile _ _ _ _ _ _ _ _ _◯ _ _ _ _ _ _◯_ _, which can transfer its stored
energy to ATP as needed.

29. The energy for making creatine phosphate and ATP comes from fuel molecules such as the simple

sugar _ ◯◯ _ _ ◯ _.

30. When additional energy is required _ _ _ _ _ ◯ _ _, stored in muscle cells, is degraded to yield glucose.

31. When muscle cells break down glucose by anaerobic metabolism, _ _ _ ◯ _ _ _ _◯ _ _ is a waste
product.

32. Muscles maintain a state of partial contraction, called ◯◯ _ _ _ _ _ _ _ ◯, an unconscious process that keeps muscles ready for activity.

33. When a motor nerve is disconnected from a muscle, the muscle loses tone and becomes ◯ _ _ _ _ ◯ _.

34. If ATP is depleted during strenuous exercise, weaker contractions and _ _ _ _ _ _ _ _ _ _ _ _ _ result.

Match the term on the left to the correct selection on the right. (Sections II and III)

35. _____ isometric

A. attachment of the muscle to the less movable bone

36. _____ insertion

B. when one muscle moves an arm and another muscle undoes the motion, the muscles are said to be this

37. _____ agonist

C. contraction in which muscle tension increases, but muscle length does not change appreciably

38. _____ fixator

D. stabilizes joints so that undesirable movement does not occur

39. _____ tendons

E. attachment of the muscle to the more movable bone

40. _____ origin

F. contraction in which muscle shortens and thickens as it contracts while the muscle tone remains the same

41. _____ antagonist

G. muscle that contracts to produce a particular action; prime mover

42. _____ antagonistic

H. skeletal muscles produce movement by pulling on these, which pull on bones

43. _____ isotonic

I. muscle that produces the opposite movement to an agonist

44. _____ synergist

J. stabilizes the origin of the prime mover so that its force is fully directed on the bone on which it inserts

Fill in the blank with the correct answer for each statement. (Section IV)

45. The _____ are circular muscles that surround the eyelids.

46. The orbicularis oris closes and protrudes the _____.

47. The _____ and the _____ muscles raise the jaw.

48. The trapezius extends the _____ and _____.

49. The _____ increases the volume of the chest cavity in inspiration.

50. The deltoid abducts the upper _____.

51. The _____ extends the forearm at the elbow.

52. The large, superficial muscle that extends the thigh and rotates the thigh medially at the hip is the

_____

53. The sartorius muscle flexes and adducts the _____

54. The tibialis dorsiflexes the _____.

55. The _____ muscles flex the leg at the knee.

56. Label the muscles in Figures 5-1 and 5-2.

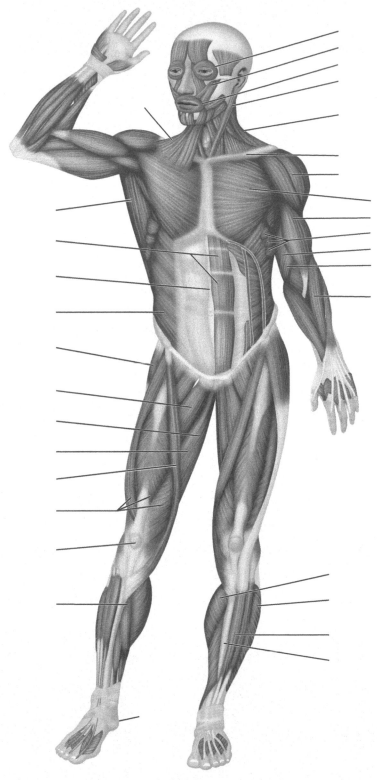

Figure 5-1

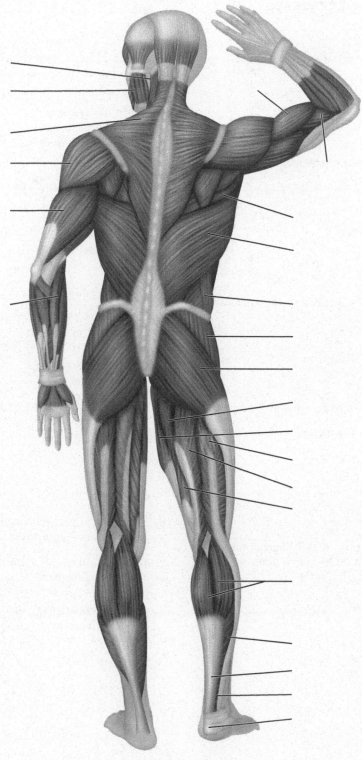

Figure 5-2

Select the correct answer.

1. Which of the following is *not* true about skeletal muscles?
   a. are attached to bone
   b. are voluntary muscles
   c. made up of connective fibers
   d. are organs

2. Individual muscle fibers are surrounded by a connective tissue covering called the _____ and are arranged in bundles called _____.
   a. endomysium; fascicles
   b. epimysium; myosin
   c. epimysium; fascicles
   d. perimysium; striations

3. Muscles are surrounded by a covering of connective tissue called the
   a. perimysium
   b. endomysium
   c. epimysium
   d. epidermis

4. Muscle is surrounded by fibrous connective tissue called _____ that merges with the tissue of the _____.
   a. epimysium; ligament
   b. fascia; ligament
   c. epimysium; tendon
   d. fascia; tendon

5. Numerous _____ in each skeletal muscle fiber provide energy for muscle contraction.
   a. nuclei
   b. mitochondria
   c. T tubules
   d. myofibrils

6. _____ are composed of small structures called muscle filaments (myofilaments) that are made of _____ threads.
   a. Muscles; plasma
   b. Myofibrils; protein
   c. Sarcomeres; protein
   d. Myofibrils; plasma

7. _____ are connected end to end to make up a myofibril.
   a. Muscle filaments
   b. Sarcomeres
   c. T tubules
   d. Fascia

8. A muscle pulls on a _____ when its fibers contract to produce _____.
   a. filament; movement
   b. bone; ATP
   c. bone; movement
   d. tendon; glucose

9. A motor nerve is made up of motor neurons that transmit _____ to muscle fibers.
   a. impulses
   b. energy
   c. motion
   d. glucose

10. _____ send signals across synapses, junctions between neurons or between a neurons and _____; muscles or glands.
   a. Muscles; filaments
   b. Nerves; effectors
   c. Neurotransmitters; filaments
   d. Neurotransmitters; effectors

Mark each statement true or false; correct the false statements to make them true.

11. _____ Acetylcholine diffuses across the synaptic cleft and combines with receptors on the surface of a muscle fiber causing depolarization.

12. _____ Depolarization of the T tubules triggers release of stored sodium ions from the endoplasmic reticulum, which bind to a protein on the myosin filament.

13. _____ VATP, which provides energy for contraction, is bound to myosin when the muscle is at rest and is split when the binding sites are exposed.

14. _____ Muscles quickly use up their store of ATP when the body undergoes strenuous exercise and must switch to the backup energy storage compound creatine phosphate.

15. _____ Glycogen is stored in muscle cells in the form of glucose which may be degraded and yields glycogen which can be broken down in cellular respiration.

16. _____ An oxygen debt develops during muscle relaxation and is paid back by a period of rapid breathing which breaks down accumulated creatine phosphate.

17. _____ Muscles maintain muscle tone as a result of continuous stimulation from nerve cells which keeps some muscle fibers in a state of contraction.

18. _____ Muscle tone is maintained by isotonic contraction in which muscles shorten and thicken as they contract.

19. _____ The attachment of the muscle to the more movable bone is its insertion, whereas attachment of the muscle to the less movable bone is called its origin.

20. _____ A muscle that produces the opposite movement, called the antagonist, is relaxed when the agonist is contracting.

21. _____ Synergists stabilize the movement of a prime mover so that its force is fully directed on the bone on which it inserts.

PART 3: ACCEPT THE CHALLENGE

1. What might happen if a body is unable to produce enough acetylcholinesterase to break down acetylcholine?

2. Based on your understanding of isotonic and isometric contraction, name (1) an isotonic and (2) an isometric exercise that you might do during a workout at the gym.

3. Describe how muscle and bone are essential parts of a lever for body movements.

Answer the questions to complete the crossword puzzle.

Muscling In

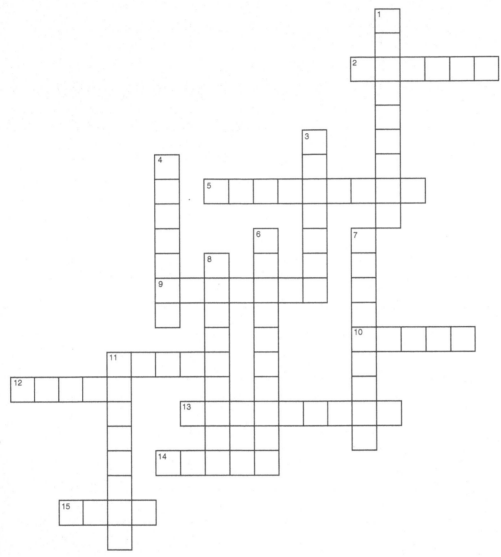

Across

2. Plantar flexes the foot
5. Smile muscle
9. Flexes and rotates the thigh
10. Brachialis flexes this joint
11. Digastric muscle opens this
12. Origin for the tibialis anterior
13. Flexes the knee and thigh
14. Insertion for the gluteus trio
15. Another name for mastication

Down

1. Raises eyebrows
3. Insertion for the deltoid
4. Abducts the upper arm
6. Whistlers need this muscle
7. Extends head and neck
8. Increases chest volume in inspiration
11. Its origin is the maxilla

6 | The Central Nervous System

LEARNING OBJECTIVES

1. Describe the main divisions of the nervous system.
2. Relate the function of neurons to their structure, and give four functions of glial cells.
3. Distinguish between nerve and tract, and between ganglion and nucleus.
4. Briefly describe the basic processes essential for neural signaling—reception, transmission, integration, and response.
5. Contrast an action potential with the resting potential of a neuron. (Describe each.)
6. Compare continuous conduction with saltatory conduction.
7. Describe the transmission of a signal across a synapse. (Draw a diagram to support your description.)
8. Describe the actions of the neurotransmitters discussed in this chapter.

9. Describe how a postsynaptic neuron integrates incoming stimuli and "decides" whether to fire.
10. Describe the structure and functions of the main parts of the brain: medulla, pons, midbrain, diencephalon (thalamus and hypothalamus), cerebellum, and cerebrum. (Label the main structures of the brain on a diagram.)
11. Describe the principal areas and functions associated with each lobe of the cerebrum and with the limbic system.
12. List two functions of the spinal cord and describe its structure.
13. Trace in sequence the structures through which signals are transmitted in a withdrawal reflex. (Draw and label a diagram of a withdrawal reflex.)
14. Describe the structures that protect the brain and spinal cord.

Match the term on the left to the correct selection on the right. (Section I)

1. _____ central

    A. part of the nervous system made up of sensory receptors and nerves

2. _____ cranial

    B. sensory receptors and nerves that regulate the internal environment

3. _____ somatic

    C. motor nerves; transmit information from the CNS to structures that must respond

4. _____ peripheral

    D. part of the nervous system that consists of the brain and spinal cord

5. _____ spinal

    E. nerves that link the brain with sensory receptors and other parts of the body

6. _____ afferent

    F. sensory receptors and nerves concerned with changes in outside environment

7. _____ efferent

    G. nerves that link the spinal cord with sensory receptors and other parts of the body

8. _____ autonomic

    H. sensory nerves; transmit messages from receptors to the CNS

Fill in the blank with the correct answer for each statement. (Section II)

9. _____ are highly specialized to receive and transmit electrical and chemical signals throughout the body.

10. The main part of the neuron, the _____, contains the nucleus and most organelles.

11. Highly branched fibers called _____ extend from the cell body and are specialized to receive _____ and transmit them to the cell body.

12. A single _____ transmits neural messages from the cell body toward another neuron, a _____, or a gland.

13. Axons may produce _____ branches and divide extensively at the distal end, forming many terminal branches that end in _____.

14. Synaptic terminals release _____, chemical compounds that transmit _____ from one neuron to another (or from a neuron to a muscle or gland).

15. Axons of many neurons of the PNS have two covers, an inner _____ and an outer _____, both of which are formed by support cells known as Schwann cells.

16. Myelin is an excellent electrical _____ that speeds the conduction of nerve impulses; neurilemma is important in growth and repair of injured _____.

17. _____ support and protect neurons, _____ with one another and with neurons, and carry out major regulatory functions.

18. _____ are star-shaped glial cells that support, protect, and communicate with neurons; _____ form insulating myelin sheaths around neurons in the CNS.

19. Ependymal cells line cavities in the CNS and help produce and circulate _____.

20. _____ multiply and move to injured, or infected, areas and remove _____ and cell debris by phagocytosis.

21. Label the parts of the neuron in Figure 6-1.

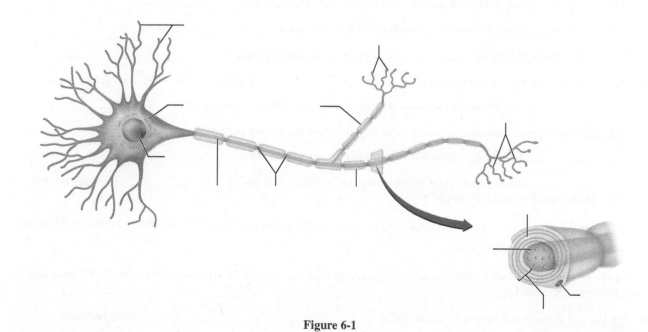

Figure 6-1

Match the following terms to the correct definitions by writing the corresponding letter in the space provided. (Sections III, IV)

A. effectors	B. ganglion	C. integration	D. nerve	E. neural signaling
F. nuclei	G. pathway	H. synapse	I. transmission	

22. _____ communication among neurons

23. _____ junction between two neurons

24. _____ group, or mass, of nerve cell bodies

25. _____ name for "ganglia" within the CNS

26. _____ large bundle of axons wrapped in connective tissue

27. _____ information from afferent neurons is sorted and interpreted; then an appropriate response is determined

28. _____ muscles and glands that cause a response to messages from the nervous system

29. _____ process of sending messages along a neuron

30. _____ designation for a "nerve" within the CNS

Fill in the blank with the correct answer for each statement. (Section V)

31. The plasma membrane is electrically _____ when one side (or pole) has a different charge from the other side.

32. The difference in electrical charge across the plasma membrane produces a _____.

33. Voltage is the force that causes _____ to flow between two points.

34. The voltage measured across the plasma membrane is referred to as the _____.

35. The membrane potential in a resting neuron (or muscle cell) is its _____.

36. Ions diffuse through specific _____ in the plasma membrane.

37. When the membrane potential becomes less negative (closer to zero) than the resting level, the membrane is

_____; it is excitatory because it brings a neuron closer to transmitting a _____.

38. When the membrane potential becomes more negative than the resting potential, the membrane is

_____; the ability of the neuron to generate a neural impulse is _____

39. _____ ion channels open when a stimulus is sufficiently strong; _____ enter the neuron
through the specific gated channels.

40. A(an) _____ (neural impulse) is generated when the voltage across the membrane is decreased to the

_____ (critical point).

Fill in the blanks to correctly complete each sentence, and then unscramble the circled letters to correctly complete the final sentence. (Section V)

41. As the action potential moves down the axon, _ _ _ _ _ ◯ _ _ _ _ ◯ _ _ _ occurs behind it.

42. The axon membrane is in a(an) _ _ _ _ _ ◯ _ _ _ _ _ _ ◯ _ _ _ _ _ period during the
millisecond in which it is depolarized.

43. During a ◯ _ ◯ _ _ _ _ _ refractory period, the axon can transmit impulses, but the threshold is higher.

44. Smooth, progressive transmission of a neural impulse is called _ ◯ _ _ _ _ _ _ _ ◯ conduction.

45. At a node of Ranvier, where the axon is not _ ◯ _ _ _ _ _ ◯ _ _, the action potential jumps to the next
node.

46. Neural transmission involving leaps from node to node is faster and requires less energy, compared with
continuous conduction; it is called _ _ _ _ _ _ _ _ _ _ conduction.

Match the term on the left to the correct selection on the right. (Section VI)

47. _____ dopamine

48. _____ GABA

49. _____ substance P

50. _____ acetylcholine

51. _____ presynaptic

52. _____ nitric oxide (NO)

53. _____ glutamate

54. _____ synaptic cleft

55. _____ postsynaptic

56. _____ endorphin

A. major excitatory neurotransmitter in the brain

B. small space that separates presynaptic and postsynaptic neurons

C. neuron that begins at a synapse

D. retrograde messenger at some synapses; transmits information from a
postsynaptic neuron to a presynaptic neuron

E. inhibits interneurons in the CNS

F. opioid made by the body, which blocks pain signals by binding to certain
receptors in the brain

G. neurotransmitter in the catecholamine group that affects mood

H. neuron that terminates at a specific synapse

I. cholinergic neurons release this neurotransmitter

J. neurotransmitter that activates pathways that transmit pain signals

Fill in the blanks with the correct answer for each statement. (Sections VI, VII)

57. Neurotransmitters are stored in synaptic terminals within small sacs called _____.

58. _____ are found on dendrites and cell bodies of postsynaptic neurons and on the _____ of muscle fibers and gland cells.

59. Neurotransmitter molecules diffuse across the _____ and combine with specific receptors on the plasma membrane of _____ cells.

60. Excess of the neurotransmitter acetylcholine is degraded by the enzyme _____.

61. In a process called _____, neurotransmitters, such as catecholamines, are actively transported back into the synaptic terminals; they are repackaged in _____ and recycled.

62. A change in membrane potential that brings the neuron closer to firing is called an _____.

63. A neurotransmitter-receptor combination that hyperpolarizes the postsynaptic membrane, taking the neuron farther away from the firing level, is called an _____

64. EPSPs may be added together, a process known as _____.

65. Each EPSP and IPSP is not an all-or-none response but is a _____ response that may be added to or subtracted from with other EPSPs and IPSPs.

66. _____ is the process of summing incoming signals; most of the process takes place in the _____.

Match the following terms to the correct definitions by writing the corresponding letter in the space provided. (Section VIII)

A. brain	B. brainstem	C. cardiac	D. gray	E. medulla
F. midbrain	G. pons	H. respiratory	I. reticular formation	J. vasomotor
K. ventricles	L. white			

67. _____ most posterior portion of the brainstem; is continuous with spinal cord

68. _____ fluid-filled spaces in the brain

69. _____ receives sensory information entering spinal cord and brainstem; influences the level of arousal

70. _____ centers in the medulla that help regulate blood pressure by controlling diameter of blood vessels

71. _____ matter of the medulla consisting mainly of nerve tracts passing between spinal cord and various portions of brain

72. _____ matter of the medulla consisting mainly of various nuclei (groups of cell bodies)

73. _____ elongated portion of the brain that looks like a stalk for the cerebrum

74. _____ bulge on the anterior surface of the brainstem; connects various parts of the brain

75. _____ shortest portion of the brainstem, extends from the pons to the diencephalon

76. _____ center in the medulla that controls heart rate

77. _____ hollow organ that is the most complex mechanism in human body

78. _____ center in the medulla that initiates and regulates breathing

Chapter **6** **The Central Nervous System**

Fill in the blanks with the correct answer for each statement. (Section VIII)

79. The cavity of the midbrain, the _____, connects the third and fourth ventricles.

80. The _____ is the part of the brain between the cerebrum and the midbrain; it has two main regions, the _____ and hypothalamus.

81. Nuclei in the thalamus serve as _____ for all sensory information (except smell) to the cerebrum; the thalamus also integrates motor information and transmits messages to _____ in the cerebrum.

82. The _____, also called the control center of the autonomic system, is positioned below the thalamus; its many nuclei help regulate _____ and reproductive behavior.

83. An important endocrine gland, the _____ is connected to the hypothalamus by a stalk of tissue.

84. The _____, a prominent X-shaped structure formed by the crossing of the optic nerves, is located in the floor of the hypothalamus.

85. The hypothalamus makes two hormones: _____, which controls the rate of water reabsorption by the kidney, and _____, which stimulates uterine contractions during childbirth and release of breast milk.

86. The hypothalamus and brainstem regulate sleep-wake cycles, or _____. The _____ in the hypothalamus is the most important of the body's biological clocks.

Unscramble and fill in these important jobs performed by the cerebellum. (Section VIII)

The cerebellum:

87. helps make _____ (vetomnme) smooth and steady.

88. helps maintain _____ (smclue eotn) and posture.

89. receives impulses from vestibular apparatus in the inner ear and uses the information to maintain _____ (milqeubiriu).

90. is important in learning _____ (tmroo islksl); plays a role in planning and coordinating _____ (alkestle) muscle actions.

91. receives information from association areas in the cerebrum and may be important in cognitive function, including _____ (eggnlaua).

Match the term on the left to the correct selection on the right. (Section VIII)

92. _____ fissures   A. sense functions (seeing, hearing, etc.) are carried out here

93. _____ cerebral cortex   B. shallow grooves that separate convolutions

94. _____ basal ganglia   C. gyri; rounded elevations of cerebrum

95. _____ lateral ventricles D. responsible for all voluntary movement and for some involuntary movement

96. _____ association areas E. thin outer layer of the cerebrum

97. _____ sulci   F. largest part of brain; controls motor activities and serves as the memory center

98. _____ sensory areas   G. paired nuclei that play an important role in movement

99. _____ motor areas

H. deep grooves that separate convolutions

100. _____ cerebrum

I. link sensory and motor areas; responsible for all intellectual activities of brain

101. _____ convolutions

J. two cavities within the cerebrum

Fill in the blanks with the correct answer for each statement. (Section VIII)

102. The _____ partially divides the cerebrum into the right and left cerebral hemispheres; the

_____ separates the cerebrum from the cerebellum.

103. The _____ is a large band of white matter that connects the right and left hemispheres.

104. The _____ connects part of the cortex (hippocampus) with the hypothalamus.

105. Fissures and sulci divide each _____ into four major lobes named after the _____ that protect them.

106. Each frontal lobe is separated from a parietal lobe by a _____.

107. The _____ of the frontal lobe is largely responsible for executive functions, such as considering consequences of behavior and problem solving.

108. _____ in the left frontal lobe directs the formation of words.

109. Sensory association areas in the _____ receive and integrate information about visual, auditory, and taste sensations from other areas of the brain, allowing persons to be aware of themselves in relation to their

_____.

110. In the occipital lobe, the area that receives visual information is the _____; the region that

_____ information is called the visual association area.

111. In the _____, the primary auditory area and the auditory association area are centers for reception and

integration of _____ messages.

Match the following terms to the correct definitions by writing the corresponding letter in the space provided. (Section VIII)

| A. amygdala | B. attachment | C. drugs | D. hippocampus |
| E. learning | F. limbic system | G. memory | H. synaptic plasticity |

112. _____ process by which we acquire information as a result of experience

113. _____ involved in the formation and retrieval of memories

114. _____ ability of the nervous system to modify synapses during learning and remembering

115. _____ prescription medicines and alcohol

116. _____ filters incoming sensory information and evaluates its importance in terms of emotional needs and survival

117. _____ group of interconnected nuclei involved in memory and in the regulation of emotion

118. _____ process by which information is encoded, stored, and retrieved

119. _____ bonding between a baby and her/his caregiver, a process involving the limbic system

120. Label the parts of the brain in Figure 6-2.

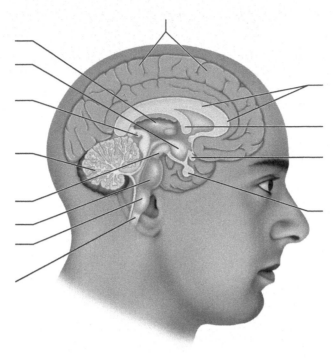

Figure 6-2

Fill in the blanks with the correct answer for each statement. (Section IX)

121. The _____ transmits information to and from the brain and controls many _____ activities of the body.

122. The spinal cord occupies the _____ of the vertebral column and is divided into regions by several deep grooves called _____.

123. The gray matter surrounds the central canal and is subdivided into _____.

124. The white matter is outside the gray matter and consists of _____ arranged in bundles, called tracts or _____.

125. Ascending tracts transmit _____ up the spinal cord to the brain.

126. _____ transmit impulses (the "decisions") from the brain back to the spinal cord to efferent nerves.

127. A reflex action is a predictable, automatic response to a specific _____ that regulates most of the internal activities of the body.

Match the following terms to the correct definitions by writing the corresponding letter in the space provided. (Section X)

A. arachnoid   **B. cerebrospinal fluid**   **C. choroid plexuses**   **D. dura mater**   **E. encephalitis**
F. meninges   **G. meningitis**   **H. pia mater**   **I. sinuses**   **J. subarachnoid space**

128. _____ outermost of the meninges; tough, double-layered membrane

129. _____ very thin membrane that adheres closely to the brain and spinal cord

130. _____ large blood vessels between two layers of dura mater

131. _____ three connective tissue layers covering the brain and spinal cord

132. _____ cushions the central nervous system

133. _____ space between the arachnoid layer and the pia mater

134. _____ second of the meninges; thin, delicate membrane

135. _____ an inflammation of the meninges, is usually caused by bacterial or viral infection

136. _____ inflammation of the brain

137. _____ clusters of capillaries which project from the pia mater into the ventricles

138. Label the parts of the spinal cord in Figure 6-3.

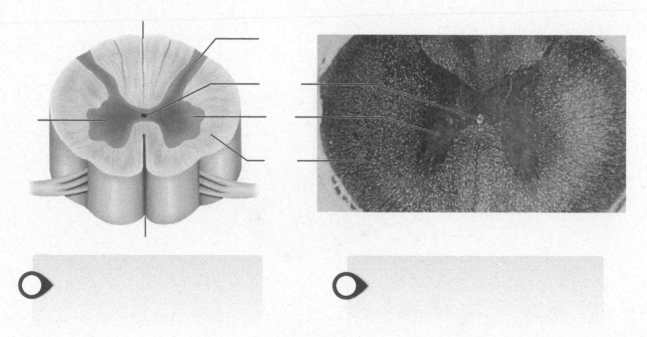

Figure 6-3

139. Label the parts of the brain in Figure 6-4.

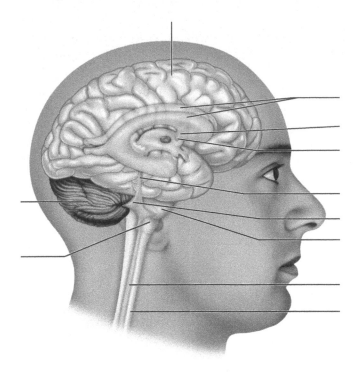

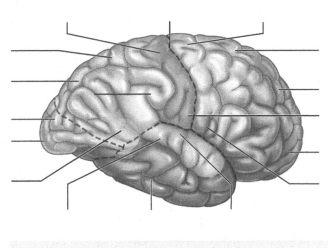

Figure 6-4

Select the correct answer.

1. The central nervous system consists of the

   _____ and _____, which
   serve as the control center of the body.
   a. brain; nerves
   b. brain; spinal cord
   c. cerebrum; medulla
   d. nerves; sensory receptors

2. The peripheral nervous system is made up of

   _____ and _____, which are
   lines of communication to and from the central
   nervous system.
   a. cerebrum; nerves
   b. brain; sensory receptors
   c. sensory receptors; nerves
   d. brain; nerves

3. Afferent, or sensory, nerves transmit messages from

   _____ to the CNS.
   a. eyes
   b. ears
   c. taste buds
   d. all of the above

4. _____ nerves transmit information back
   from the CNS to the structures that must respond.
   a. Sensory
   b. Motor
   c. Efferent
   d. b and c

5. Which of the following is not a function of glial
   cells?
   a. surround and protect cranial nerves
   b. support and protect neurons
   c. carry out major regulatory functions
   d. communicate with one another

6. The correct sequential process for neural signaling is
   a. response, transmission, integration, actual
      response, transmission
   b. reception, transmission, integration, transmission,
      actual response
   c. reception, transmission, actual response,
      transmission, integration
   d. transmission, response, transmission, response,
      integration

7. The gradients that determine the resting potential

   are maintained by _____ in the plasma
   membrane.
   a. chloride ions
   b. chloride-potassium pumps
   c. sodium-potassium pumps
   d. sodium ion pumps

8. Neurons signal other cells with neurotransmitters

   that bind with _____ on postsynaptic
   neurons.
   a. axons
   b. brain cells
   c. receptors
   d. sodium ions

9. The main divisions of the brain are the
   a. medulla, pons, midbrain, diencephalon,
      cerebellum, and cerebrum
   b. pons, midbrain, cerebrum, and cerebellum
   c. diencephalon, medulla, midbrain, cerebrum, and
      spinal cord
   d. medulla, midbrain, diencephalon, cerebellum,
      and spinal cord

10. The elongated portion of the brain, the brainstem, is
    made up of all of the following except
    a. medulla
    b. thalamus
    c. midbrain
    d. pons

11. Which of the following is not true concerning the
    medulla?
    a. acts as center for audio reflexes
    b. initiates breathing
    c. helps regulate blood pressure
    d. controls heart rate

12. The midbrain contains centers for
    a. cardiac and respiratory functions
    b. vomiting an sneezing reflexes
    c. respiration and sleep functions
    d. visual and audio reflexes

13. Which of the following is not a function of the
    hypothalamus?
    a. helps regulate homeostasis
    b. manufactures antidiuretic hormone
    c. helps regulate reproduction
    d. relays sensory information to the cerebrum

14. The cerebellum is responsible for
    a. coordination of movements
    b. storing sensory memories
    c. producing oxytocin
    d. all of the above

15. The cerebrum performs all of the following functions except
    a. interprets sensory messages
    b. maintains muscle tone
    c. controls voluntary movement
    d. links sensory and motor areas

Mark each statement true or false; correct false statements to make them true.

16. _____ The hypothalamus, along with the brainstem, regulates sleep-wake cycles, or circadian rhythms.

17. _____ The convolutions of the cerebellum are separated by shallow grooves called fissures and by deep grooves called sulci.

18. _____ A large band of gray matter, the fornix, connects the right and left hemispheres.

19. _____ Broca's area in the left frontal lobe directs the formation of words.

20. _____ The limbic system plays a role in memory, the regulation of emotion, sexual behavior, and biological rhythms.

21. _____ The amygdala filters incoming sensory information and evaluates its importance in terms of emotional needs and survival.

22. _____ Synaptic plasticity refers to the ability of the nervous system to modify synapses when dopamine concentration is low.

23. _____ Reflex actions are unpredictable, automatic responses to an unspecified stimulus.

24. _____ The spinal cord transmits information to and from the brain and controls many reflex activities of the body.

25. _____ The five steps of the reflex pathway are reception of stimulus, transmission of information to CNS, integration, transmission of information from the CNS to a muscle, and actual response.

PART 3: ACCEPT THE CHALLENGE

1. How might exercise and physical activity improve mood? How might these activities relieve pain?

2. What part of your brain allows you to consciously control your breathing while meditating and override involuntary respiration?

3. How are pathways in the spinal column affected when the spinal cord is damaged and paralysis occurs?

THE PUZZLE

Find and circle the following words from Chapter 6. Words may be found from top to bottom, bottom to top, right to left, left to right, and diagonally.

```
C F D U V M X D B X Z P E B U E Y O N P N E C P C U N H N H
A I L H F O F B C C G G A H V G A I R K I S G Z Y T B P Y Y
E H L Y N H A V Y N L D O O H S W U J D R P R N I D W Q C U
K E L P K E P M R P C Z M C T M Y H C O O A A I A D B R Q J
X M A O Z I M F Y T W J K R N A O M N Q A N N X E B O E J O
H K H T A V G O V G G Z O J L S F X A F V Y X T U K M K X J
O A X H V L N C V X D C E T D V V Q X L U S A Q O F W T A V
P K G A B W F K M G Y A K H T E Z M O P Y Q H C L A P H A O
W I I L M R I I G T U Q L J S N X W N F F G M Z H A Q G R A
K N E A A Z O B E Q K J C A B T T M K Q O C C I P I T A L C
T T I M A R P S H Z C G H C W R N E V W Z C Z Y Q C Q C N T
F E I U H R Y K N J M E Y T E I C Z C L H Y A C X B G Y Z Y
A G Q S A P L G S N O P X S X C W I E K G A N G L I O N F S
R R F O V I Q I P Q K T P L C L N R M A P C D E P J C K I A
Q A V X H J M M X N H U P R L E F A B H V M J K Y L A D O G
U T X I I E I K X F I R G R E F A L A U R C E R E B R U M O
Z I U V W N G G J G R H L J G R E O R F C K P M H U E P L K
U O N K O G R A Q A V O P G B X N P E V I Y B C E I E R Y Q
Y N S W Q G G O K T T B A R T T A E C R J J U H Y P M R W S
T D B Z U Z S U F T O K B X O X X D E S A X L V Z C U E K Z
N I O F H H A K K A E L S Y E D I L P G B R A I N F L I F X
K C L F D P J Q O X Y D E H M E N R T W A E V H Y W L N H H
V M R A M B E X G I M R A B O Y G E O S L I S Z Z O E D X P
X E T K L C G Z T G L U L I C V V T R V L Y K V E C B D W A
B F M H C J L X T Y Z B X U I J Q V S R U S S O L P E O X R
M U P C N D X E M Z P X Y L V X M V R W D E H T X B R L O I
O C C M P X O H P R G W E H L D F W B E E L W X J C E G D E
Z H Q N X T S J K R Z T G R Z E X I Q C M N O F K B C D Q T
L F W O F F G U C B O O L F N G O G H S F P K T C Z P X C A
T N N Y L D F S K A N E U R O T R A N S M I T T E R X N O L
```

amygdala	hypothalamus
astrocytes	integration
axon	medulla
brain	occipital
cerebellum	neurotransmitter
cerebrum	parietal
depolarize	pons
endorphin	receptors
fornix	synapse
ganglion	ventricle

7 The Peripheral Nervous System

LEARNING OBJECTIVES

1. Describe the components of the somatic division of the peripheral nervous system (PNS).
2. List the cranial nerves and give the functions of each.
3. Describe the function and structure of a typical spinal nerve.
4. Name and describe the major plexuses.
5. Contrast the autonomic division with the somatic division.
6. Describe a reflex pathway in the autonomic division.
7. Contrast the sympathetic system with the parasympathetic system.
8. Compare the effects of sympathetic and parasympathetic stimulation on specific organs such as the heart and the digestive tract.

PART 1: LEARN THE TERMS

Match the term on the left to the correct selection on the right. (Section I)

1. _____ afferent

2. _____ cranial

3. _____ somatic

4. _____ efferent

5. _____ autonomic

6. _____ spinal

7. _____ sensory

8. _____ peripheral

A. receptors that react to changes in the outside world

B. neurons that signal muscles and glands to respond

C. nervous system made up of sensory receptors, nerves that link sensory receptors with the central nervous system (CNS), and nerves that link the CNS with effectors

D. nerves that link brain with sensory receptors and muscles; 12 pairs

E. division of the PNS that keeps the body in adjustment with the outside world

F. nerves that link spinal cord with various structures; 31 pairs

G. neurons that keep the CNS informed of changes in the outside world

H. division of the PNS with nerves and receptors that maintain internal balance

Unscramble each spinal nerve and match it to its correct description. (Section I)

9. _____ arlmub   A. five pairs of nerves, numbered S1 to S5

10. _____ gyoleaccc   B. eight pairs of nerves, numbered C1 to C8

11. _____ raslca   C. 12 pairs of nerves, numbered T1 to T12

12. _____ rchicato   D. five pairs of nerves, numbered L1 to L5

13. _____ vreclaic   E. just one pair of nerves

Fill in the blank with the correct answer for each statement. (Section I)

14. The _____ consists only of afferent (sensory) fibers that transmit information from the sensory

     receptors to the _____.

15. The _____ is located just before the dorsal root joins the spinal cord; it consists of the

     _____ of the sensory neurons.

16. The _____ consists only of efferent (motor) fibers leaving the spinal cord.

17. Dorsal and ventral roots join to form a _____, which divides into _____ just after leaving
the vertebral column.

18. The dorsal (posterior) branch of each nerve supplies the muscles and skin of the _____ part of the
body in that region.

19. The ventral (anterior) branch innervates the _____ and lateral body trunk in that area, as well as the

     _____.

20. The _____ of several spinal nerves interconnect and form networks called plexuses; each plexus is a

     tangled network of fibers from all of the _____ involved.

Match the following terms to the correct definitions by writing the corresponding letter in the space provided.
(Section I)

A. brachial   B. cervical   C. femoral   D. lumbar
E. phrenic   F. sacral   G. sciatic   H. ulnar

21. _____ plexus that supplies the lower abdominal wall, thigh, and external genital structures

22. _____ plexus that supplies the buttock, thigh, leg, and foot

23. _____ nerve that exits from cervical plexus and transmits impulses to the diaphragm

24. _____ plexus that supplies the lower part of the shoulder, the arm, and the hand

25. _____ main branch of the sacral plexus; largest nerve in the body

26. _____ largest nerve arising from the lumbar plexus

27. _____ nerve that arises from the brachial plexus; "funny bone"

28. _____ plexus that sends information to the skin and muscles of part of the head, neck, and upper shoulders

Fill in the blanks with the correct answer for each statement. (Section II)

29. The autonomic division works to maintain _____ within the body by acting on smooth muscle, _____, and glands.

30. The _____ portion of the autonomic division is subdivided into sympathetic and _____ systems.

31. The _____ system prepares the body for action and is most active during _____ times.

32. Neurons of the sympathetic system emerge from the _____ and lumbar regions of the _____.

33. Sympathetic neurons pass through the _____ branch and then pass into the _____ of the paravertebral sympathetic ganglion chain.

34. Some of the first efferent neurons do not end in the ganglia of the paravertebral chain; they pass on to _____ ganglia located in the abdomen.

35. The first efferent neurons are referred to as _____ neurons; they release the neurotransmitter _____ and are referred to as cholinergic neurons.

36. The second efferent neurons are _____ neurons. The postganglionic neurons release norepinephrine and are referred to as _____ neurons.

Match the following terms to the correct definitions by writing the corresponding letter in the space provided. (Section II)

A. acetylcholine   **B. adrenergic**   **C. cholinergic**   **D. muscarinic**   **E. nicotinic**
F. opposite   **G. parasympathetic**   **H. pelvic**   **I. terminal ganglia**   **J. vagus**

37. _____ located near or within the walls of the organs they innervate

38. _____ system that helps return the body to resting conditions; conserves and restores energy

39. _____ sympathetic and parasympathetic nerves have this effect on many organs

40. _____ nerve that innervates many thoracic and abdominal organs

41. _____ receptors are activated when acetylcholine binds with them

42. _____ norepinephrine binds to this receptor

43. _____ parasympathetic nerves that emerge from the sacral region form these nerves

44. _____ receptors located on postganglionic neurons in all autonomic ganglia

45. _____ receptors found on cardiac muscle fibers, smooth muscle fibers, and gland cells

46. _____ preganglionic and postganglionic fibers of parasympathetic system release this neurotransmitter

47. Label the spinal cord and nerves in Figure 7-1.

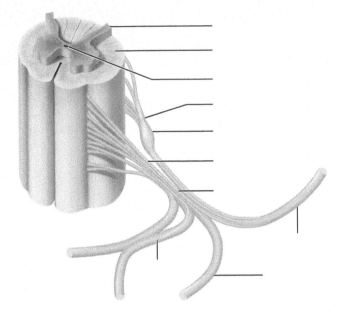

Figure 7-1

PART 2

1. The PNS is made up of
   a. nerves that link sensory receptors with the central nervous system
   b. sensory receptors
   c. nerves that link the CNS with effectors
   d. all of the above

2. The afferent and efferent neurons of the somatic division, along with neurons of the autonomic division, make up the
   a. cranial and spinal nerves
   b. vagus and pelvic nerves
   c. brain and spinal column
   d. none of the above

3. Cranial nerves transmit orders in the form of neural signals from the brain to
   a. sensory receptors
   b. muscles and glands
   c. spinal nerves
   d. all of the above

4. There are 12 pairs of _____ spinal nerves and 5 pairs of _____ spinal nerves.
   a. cervical; thoracic
   b. thoracic; lumbar
   c. lumbar; cervical
   d. sacral; lumbar

5. Each spinal _____ consists of the cell bodies of sensory neurons.
   a. neuron
   b. ganglion
   c. cord
   d. plexus

6. Dorsal and ventral roots join to form a

   _____
   a. ganglion
   b. spinal cord
   c. spinal nerve
   d. plexus

7. The phrenic nerve, which exits from the cervical

   plexus, transmits impulses to the _____.
   a. brain
   b. heart
   c. diaphragm
   d. lungs

8. Two of the nerves that emerge from the brachial plexus are the _____ and the _____

   a. ulnar; radial
   b. ulnar; vagus
   c. vagus; radial
   d. sciatic; radial

9. The largest nerve in the body, the _____ nerve, can be compressed (pinched) by a herniated disk in the lower back resulting in numbness in the leg and pain that radiates from the hip down through the leg.

   a. sciatic
   b. femoral
   c. vagus
   d. radial

Mark each statement true or false; correct false statements to make them true.

10. _____ The somatic division works to keep the body in adjustment with the outside world; the autonomic division works to maintain homeostasis within the body.

11. _____ The efferent portion of the somatic division is subdivided into sympathetic and parasympathetic systems.

12. _____ In the autonomic division *two* afferent neurons are found between the PNS and the muscle or gland it innervates.

13. _____ When muscarinic receptors are activated, the effect can be excitatory or inhibitory depending on the effector.

14. _____ Nicotinic receptors are activated by acetylcholine released from both sympathetic and parasympathetic preganglionic neurons.

15. _____ Beta blockers are antagonistic drugs that block acetylcholine.

16. _____ When norepinephrine binds to beta receptors in cardiac muscle, the heart beats faster and stronger.

PART 3: ACCEPT THE CHALLENGE

1. Describe which system of the autonomic division would be dominant while you are driving your car in a downpour? Which autonomic division would become dominant after you pull into a parking lot to rest?

2. How would messages from the brain be affected if the spinal cord became damaged?

Answer the questions to complete the crossword puzzle.

You've Got Nerve

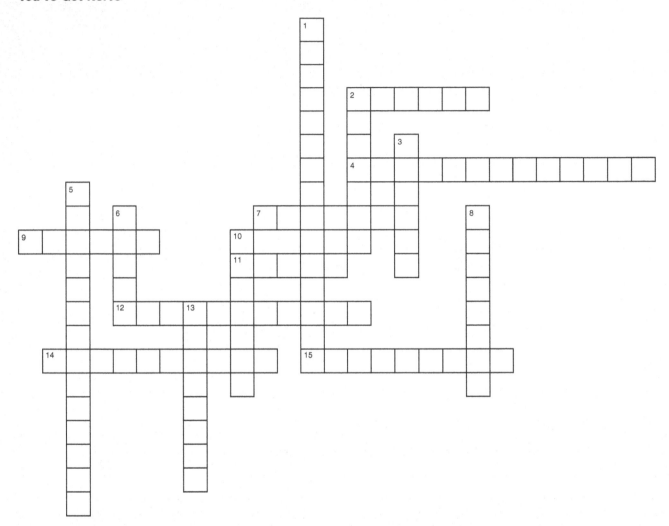

Across

2. plexus that supplies feet
4. preganglionic neuron releases this
7. nerve that links brain with sensory receptors and muscles
9. root made up of sensory fibers
11. pairs of cervical spinal nerves
12. system that prepares you for action
14. the "P" in PNS
15. one pair of this spinal nerve

Down

1. system most active during rest time
2. division that includes sensory receptors, afferent neurons, and efferent neurons
3. pathway in the autonomic division
5. an adrenergic neuron releases this
6. parasympathetic nerve that drops heart rate
8. plexus that serves the head
10. root consists of motor fibers
13. ventral branches form these

8 The Sense Organs

CHAPTER GUIDE

I. Sensory receptors transduce the energy of a stimulus into electrical signals
    A. Sensory receptors produce receptor potentials
    B. We can differentiate between seeing a dog and tasting a cookie
    C. Sensory receptors adapt to stimuli
    D. The mind constructs sensory perceptions
II. Sensory receptors respond to different types of energy
III. The eye contains photoreceptors
    A. The eye is well protected
    B. The eye is enclosed by three specialized tissue layers
    C. The eyes form a sharp image
    D. The retina contains light-sensitive rods and cones
    E. The optic nerves transmit signals to the brain

IV. The ear functions in hearing and equilibrium
    A. The outer ear conducts sound waves to the middle ear
    B. The middle ear amplifies sound waves
    C. The inner ear contains mechanoreceptors
        1. The cochlea contains the receptors for hearing
        2. Sounds differ in pitch, loudness, and quality
    D. The vestibule and semicircular canals help maintain equilibrium
V. Chemoreceptors sense smell and taste
    A. Chemoreceptors in the nasal cavity sense odorants
    B. Taste buds detect dissolved food molecules
VI. The general senses are widespread through the body
    A. Tactile receptors are located in the skin
    B. Temperature receptors are nerve endings
    C. Pain sensation is a protective mechanism
    D. Proprioceptors inform us of our position

LEARNING OBJECTIVES

1. Describe how a sensory receptor functions. (Include sensory reception, energy transduction, receptor potential, sensory adaptation, and perception.)
2. Classify sensory receptors according to the type of energy they transduce.
3. Describe the anatomy of the eye and give the function of each structure. (Include a description of the visual pathway.)
4. Describe the structures and functions of the three major parts of the ear.
5. Trace the transmission of sound through the ear.
6. Describe the functions of the vestibule and semicircular canals.
7. Compare the receptors of smell and taste.
8. Describe the tactile receptors and temperature receptors.
9. Describe the process of pain perception and explain the basis of phantom and referred pain.
10. Locate proprioceptors in the body and describe their functions.

PART 1: LEARN THE TERMS

Fill in the blanks with the correct answer for each statement. (Section I)

1. A _____ is any internal or external change we detect in our environment.

2. We detect stimuli through our _____ receptors, which convert (transduce) the energy of a stimulus to _____ energy.

3. Sensory receptors, along with other types of cells, make up complex _____: our eyes, ears, nose, and _____.

4. A sensory receptor absorbs a small amount of energy from some stimulus in the environment and converts it into electrical energy, a process known as _____.

5. A change in membrane potential occurs and produces a _____, a depolarization or hyperpolarization of the membrane, which may generate action potentials in a sensory neuron.

6. The sensory neuron transmits signals to the CNS where _____ takes place.

7. A receptor potential is a _____, meaning that the extent of change depends on the energy of the stimulus.

8. Each type of sensory receptor normally responds to only one type of _____; each receptor is connected by _____ to a particular area of the brain.

9. The brain recognizes the type of stimulus it receives from a particular sensory receptor and _____ the incoming sensory message.

10. The intensity of a stimulus is coded by the frequency of _____ transmitted by a given fiber.

11. A painful backache would involve a _____ frequency of action potentials compared with a minor scratch on the skin.

12. Over time a response to a continued, constant stimulus decreases; sensory _____ is a decrease in frequency of action potentials in a sensory neuron even though the stimulus is maintained.

13. Sensory _____ is the process of selecting, interpreting, and organizing sensory information.

Unscramble the sensory receptors below and match them to their correct description. (Section II)

14. _____ ocrmpehrettreo   A. transduces light energy

15. _____ creehcneptmoaro   B. responds to heat and cold

16. _____ trheoceoprpot   C. transduces chemical compounds

17. _____ etomrhcepcoer   D. responds to pain

18. _____ pcienctoro   E. transduces mechanical energy (touch, pressure, or gravity)

Match the following terms to the correct definitions by writing the corresponding letter in the space provided. (Section III)

A. binocular	B. choroid	C. conjunctiva	D. cornea	E. eye
F. iris	G. lacrimal	H. pupil	I. sclera	J. tears

19. _____ tough, fibrous tissue; the "white of the eye"

20. _____ gland that produces tears

21. _____ keep eyes moist and free of dust

22. _____ its blood vessels nourish the retina

23. _____ regulates the amount of light entering eye

24. _____ vision helps us judge distances and depth

25. _____ opening in the center of circular muscles of the iris

26. _____ transparent layer that covers the iris and pupil

27. _____ organ of vision

28. _____ mucous membrane that covers sclera; lines inner layer of eyelid

Fill in the blanks with the correct answer for each statement. (Section III)

29. The anterior cavity between the cornea and the lens is filled with a watery substance called the _____.

30. The larger posterior cavity between the lens and the retina is filled with a viscous fluid called the

_____.

31. The iris regulates the amount of _____ entering the eye; it is composed of two mutually

_____ sets of smooth muscle fibers.

32. The _____, an adjustable, transparent, elastic ball lying just behind the iris, refracts (bends) the light

rays coming in and brings them to a focus on the _____.

33. Six _____ control eye movement by positioning the eyeball with coordinated and precise actions.

34. The eye has the ability to change focus for near or far vision by changing the shape of the lens; this is called the

power of _____ and is a function of the ciliary muscle.

35. The lens is attached to the ciliary muscles by tiny fibers that make up the _____.

36. The _____ are glandlike folds that project toward the lens and secrete the aqueous humor.

Match the term on the left to the correct selection on the right. (Section III)

37. _____ retina   A. region of sharpest vision; greatest concentration of cones

38. _____ cones   B. lateral geniculate nucleus controls which information is sent here

39. _____ rods   C. X-shaped structure where optic nerves cross the floor of the hypothalamus

40. _____ fovea   D. breakdown of this pigment leads to transduction of light and transmission of
                                  neural signals

41. _____ ganglion   E. responsible for color vision and vision during daylight

42. _____ optic nerve   F. transmits touch and pain information from eye to brain

43. _____ bipolar   G. innermost layer of eye, contains the photoreceptors

44. _____ optic chiasm   H. axons of ganglion cells across retina surface unite to form this

45. _____ rhodopsin   I. bipolar cells make synaptic contact with these cells

46. _____ optic disk   J. responsible mainly for vision in dim light or darkness

47. _____ primary visual cortex   K. photoreceptors synapse on these cells

48. _____ trigeminal nerve   L. area where the optic nerve passes out of the eyeball; blind spot

49. Label the parts of the eye in Figure 8-1.

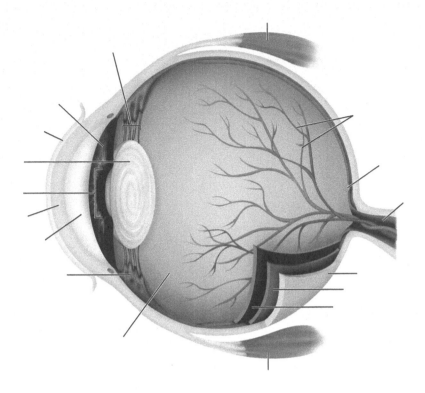

Figure 8-1

Fill in the blanks with the correct answer for each statement. (Section IV)

50. The _____ includes the visible part on the head and the canal connecting with the middle ear.

51. The _____ projects from the side of the head and surrounds the ear canal.

52. The ear canal, called the _____, leads to the middle ear.

53. The lining of the ear canal contains ceruminous _____ that secrete earwax, or _____, which helps protect the lining of the canal from infection.

54. The _____, or eardrum, separates the middle ear from the external ear.

55. The middle ear is a small, moist cavity in the _____ bone containing air and three small bones,

    or _____.

56. Air pressure is equalized on both sides of the tympanic membrane by the _____, which connects the

    _____ and the nasopharynx.

57. The three auditory ossicles, the _____, _____, and _____ form a chain from the tympanic membrane to the oval window.

58. When _____ vibrate the tympanic membrane, the auditory ossicles act as three interconnected levers to help _____ these vibrations.

59. The inner ear contains _____ that convert sound waves to nerve impulses and receptors that maintain _____.

60. The inner ear is a bony labyrinth composed of three compartments: the _____, which lies next to the oval window, the cochlea, and the _____.

61. The bony labyrinth contains _____, a fluid that surrounds the membranous labyrinth; the membranous labyrinth contains a fluid called _____.

62. Perilymph and endolymph carry _____ through the canal system of the inner ear.

Match the following terms to the correct definitions by writing the corresponding letter in the space provided. (Section IV)

| A. basilar membrane | B. cochlea | C. cochlear duct | D. cochlear nerve | E. glutamate |
| F. hair cells | G. organ of Corti | H. round window | I. stereocilia | J. vestibular |

63. _____ arranged in rows in the cochlea

64. _____ sound receptor contained in cochlea

65. _____ canal connected to tympanic canal at apex of cochlea

66. _____ neurotransmitter; binds to receptors on sensory neurons that synapse on each hair cell

67. _____ snail-shaped portion of inner ear; consists of three separated canals

68. _____ middle canal; contains organ of Corti

69. _____ tiny projections that extend into the cochlear duct

70. _____ transmits messages to the brain

71. _____ separates the cochlear duct from the tympanic canal; hair cells rest here

72. _____ membrane at the end of the tympanic canal

Fill in the blanks with the correct answer for each statement. (Section IV)

73. Pitch depends on _____ of sound waves, or number of _____ per second, and is expressed as hertz (Hz).

74. The _____ infers the pitch of a sound from the particular hair cells that are stimulated.

75. Loud sounds cause waves of greater _____.

76. Variations in the _____ of sound depend on the number and kinds of overtones, or harmonics, produced.

77. The _____ and _____ canals contain receptor cells that transmit information about the position of the body.

78. Two saclike chambers, the _____, and the _____, house gravity detectors in the form of small calcium carbonate ear stones called _____.

79. Each receptor cell has a group of hair cells that are surrounded at the tips by a gelatinous mass called a

_____

80. The three semicircular canals provide information about turning movements, referred to as _____.

81. A small, bulblike enlargement, the _____, is located at one of the openings of each canal into the utricle; a clump of hair cells called a _____ lies within each ampulla.

82. As the position of the head changes, _____ move in relation to the fluid in the canals and are stimulated by its flow; this stimulation causes an awareness of _____.

83. Responses of the sensory cells in the semicircular canals are transmitted to the vestibular nerve, which joins the cochlear nerve to form the _____ nerve.

84. Label the parts of the ear in Figure 8-2.

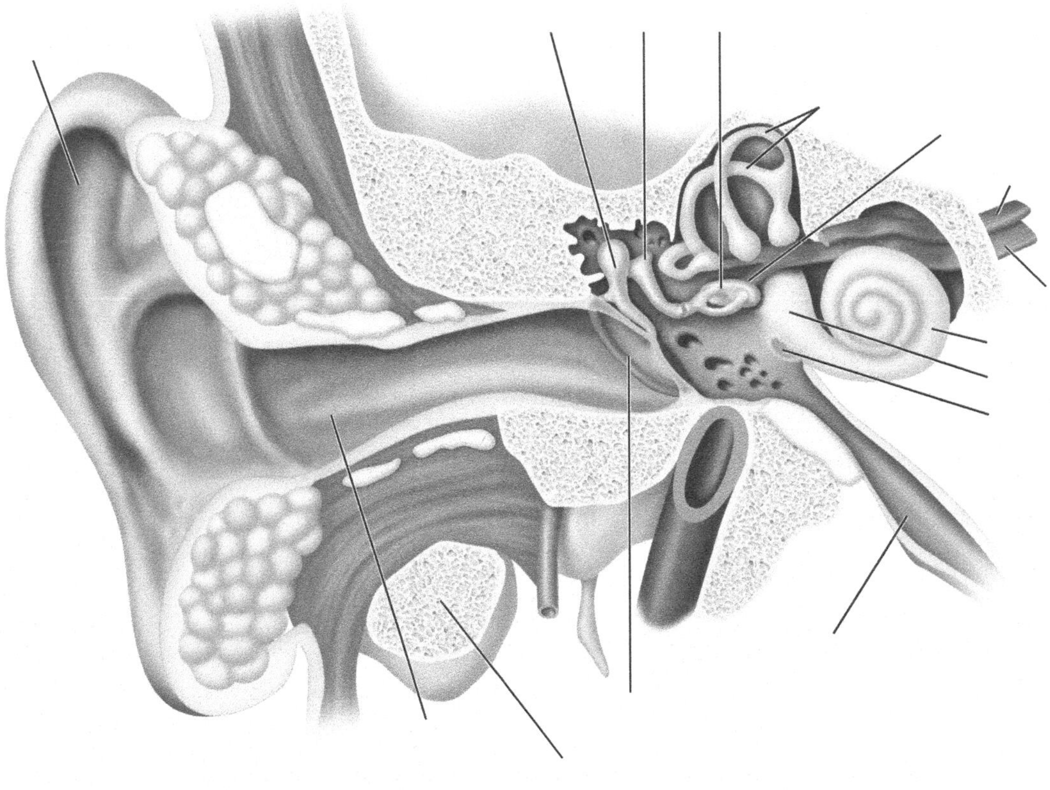

Figure 8-2

Match the term on the left to the correct selection on the right. (Section V)

85. _____ olfactory nerve   A. lines upper part of the nasal cavity

86. _____ papillae   B. detect chemical substances in air, food, and water

87. _____ umami   C. transmits odors detected by olfactory epithelium

88. _____ taste receptors   D. sense of taste carried out by taste buds

89. _____ olfaction   E. tiny elevations on the tongue that contain taste buds

90. _____ chemoreceptors   F. chemical substances that can be smelled

91. _____ smell   G. taste of savoriness

92. _____ olfactory epithelium   H. paired with taste it stimulates appetite and digestive juices

93. _____ tastes   I. oval epithelial capsule with about 100 taste receptor cells

94. _____ taste bud   J. sense of smell

95. _____ odorants   K. detect chemical substances dissolved in saliva

96. _____ gustation   L. sweet, salty, bitter, sour, and umami

Fill in the blanks with the correct answer for each statement. (Section VI)

97. The general senses are mostly _____ that respond to touch, pressure, vibration, changes in temperature, and muscle stretch; _____ sense pain.

98. Mechanoreceptors that are free _____ detect touch and pressure when stimulated by objects that contact the body surface.

99. Thousands of more specialized _____ receptors, also located in the skin, sense light touch and pressure, heavy and continuous touch and pressure, and deep pressure.

100. _____, free nerve endings that detect temperature change, are especially concentrated in the _____ and mouth.

101. Thermoreceptors in the _____ detect internal changes in temperature and receive and integrate information from thermoreceptors on the body surface.

102. Nociceptors are free nerve endings of certain _____ neurons found in almost every tissue; they respond to temperature extremes and strong tactile _____

103. Sensory neurons release _____ and several other neurotransmitters, including substance P, which stimulate neurons in the spinal cord to transmit pain signals to the brain.

104. The principal ascending pain pathway is the _____ tract, which transmits signals to the _____, where pain perception begins.

105. The body makes _____, including endorphins and enkephalins, for _____, or pain control.

106. Opiates inhibit the release of _____ to decrease transmission of pain signals up the spinal cord.

107. For years after an amputation, a patient may feel _____ in the missing limb because the brain remembers the message from the nerve during the amputation.

Fill in the blanks to correctly complete each sentence, and then unscramble the circled letters to correctly complete the final sentence. (Section V)

108. _ _ _ ◯ _ _ _ _ _ _ _ ◯ _ _ help maintain the position of the body and its parts.

109. Muscle spindles detect _ _ ◯ _ _ _ movement.

110. Golgi tendon organs determine _ ◯ _ _ _ _ _ in the tendons that attach muscle to bone.

111. _ ◯ _ ◯ _ receptors detect movement in ligaments.

112. The brain coordinates information from proprioceptors with input from the inner ear to maintain

_ _ _ ◯ _ _ _ _ ◯ _ _ and coordination of muscular activities.

113. Our conscious awareness of body _ _ _ _ _ _ _ _ and movement is called kinesthetic sense.

PART 2: ASSESS YOUR UNDERSTANDING

Select the correct answer.

1. Sensory receptors transduce the energy of a stimulus

   into _____
   a. pressure
   b. electrical signals
   c. reflexes
   d. none of the above

2. Which of the following is *not* involved in sensory processing
   a. energy is transduced
   b. change in membrane potential occurs
   c. receptor potential generates action potentials
   d. integration takes place in sensory neuron

3. The brain interprets sensations by converting them to

   _____ of the stimuli received by our sensory receptors.
   a. memories
   b. perceptions
   c. detectors
   d. reflections

4. _____ transduce touch, pressure, gravity, stretching, and movement directly into electrical signals.
   a. mechanoreceptors
   b. chemoreceptors
   c. nociceptors
   d. photoreceptors

5. Which sensory receptors would respond if you spilled hot coffee in your lap?
   a. mechanoreceptors and thermoreceptors
   b. photoreceptor and nociceptors
   c. thermoreceptors and nociceptors
   d. chemoreceptors and thermoreceptors

6. Which of the following is not a part of the eyeball?
   a. cornea
   b. iris
   c. cochlea
   d. retina

7. The _____ layer of the eyeball contains blood vessels that nourish the retina.
   a. sclera
   b. conjunctiva
   c. cornea
   d. choroid

8. An abnormal accumulation of _____ increases the intraocular pressure in the eye; this can damage the retina and optic nerve, resulting in glaucoma.
   a. vitreous humor
   b. blood
   c. aqueous humor
   d. tears

9. Which part of the eye refracts light rays coming into the eye to bring them to a focus on the retina?
   a. lens
   b. iris
   c. pupil
   d. conjunctiva

10. Which is true concerning the fovea?
    a. Cones are most concentrated here.
    b. It is the region of sharpest vision.
    c. both a and b
    d. none of the above

11. Photoreceptors (rods and cones) synapse on

_____ cells, which make synaptic

contact with _____ cells.
   a. ganglion; nerve
   b. bipolar; ganglion
   c. nerve; bipolar
   d. ganglion; bipolar

12. What part of the ear contains sensory receptors for sound waves and for maintaining the equilibrium of the body?
   a. outer ear
   b. middle ear
   c. inner ear
   d. tympanic membrane

Mark each statement true or false; correct false statements to make them true.

13. _____ The lining of the external auditory meatus contains ceruminous glands that secrete earwax, or cerumen.

14. _____ Incoming sound waves cause the tympanic membrane to vibrate, transmitting sound waves into the inner ear.

15. _____ The eustachian tube connects the middle ear and the nasopharynx; it equalizes the air pressure on both sides of the oval window.

16. _____ A very small movement in the malleus causes a larger movement in the incus and a very large movement in the stapes.

17. _____ The middle ear is a bony labyrinth that contains chemoreceptors that convert sound waves to nerve impulses.

18. _____ Each organ of Corti, located in the cochlea, contains sensory cells that respond to sound waves by stimulating the cochlear nerve.

19. _____ Depolarization of hair cells on the basilar membrane may cause a receptor potential to be generated.

20. _____ Exposure to heavily amplified music or other high-intensity sound damages the hair cells of the organ of Corti.

21. _____ Chemoreceptors cells are stimulated by odorants that dissolve in the mucus on the surface of the tongue.

22. _____ Taste receptors, found in the taste buds of the tongue, detect chemical substances dissolved in saliva.

23. _____ Four main tastes are recognized: sweet, sour, salty, and bitter.

24. _____ Thermoreceptors in the hypothalamus detect internal changes in temperature, and receive and integrate information from thermoreceptors on the body surface.

25. _____ The spinothalamic tract transmits signals to the cerebrum, where pain perception begins.

26. _____ The brain coordinates information from proprioceptors with input from the vestibule and semicircular canals in the inner ear to maintain equilibrium and coordination of muscular activities.

PART 3: ACCEPT THE CHALLENGE

1. Explain how sensory adaptation can be an evolutionary advantage?

2. How do eyeglasses correct vision?

3. What causes you to feel dizzy and stagger after you get off a wildly spinning carnival ride?

Find and circle the following words from Chapter 8. Words may be found from top to bottom, bottom to top, right to left, left to right, and diagonally.

```
K S Q S A G I T X F H Z K A Q J V U I Y H R B M M O A U N H
I N E G F E I C A V D F T R O M U H S U O E U Q A N F T C S
G Y L B B O N N K F E V O D X A W U S K B W F Z Y Z B N X H
R J U R E Z V F R L U D Q X Z N I O N Q Z J H D M Q O L A S
B W B H K D B E H Q R G P U G J S F R H Q E H Y I B O U I T
G U I T Q S J Z A V G Y I B L K R A N I T E R R R M H A L I
E R T I X Z I L Q D X Z K Q R U D B E S H I Y U L H N V I V
M U S P Z D L R E D S N H K D A M O T L J K N E K U U Z C U
G Q E Y I F G O I T U J B C N Y V V D A L Q N T G J L E O H
S K V H K S I N C U S D R U F B P O A N Z S C L Y I Q P E L
X S Z N O B Z B Q E K L V Y V E U K K L D L U Y K E X I R U
L C S W X C F M W N O I T A T S U G V D V T O B M R J W E S
L I S Z U N Y U W W C O P J H C O V T E A V N D I E H M T J
A X Q M T N E Y R E K M Q I J B C H V M U U U I Z E W G S D
B Y C A R E L Q V Z R L I Z V R A I A R A X L B A D M W C M
E Z D K I M P G M Y E Q M T F J X T A J D N F W N R C Z Z U
Y H Q T C S H R C H E M O R E C E P T O R Q A C E R B L Y F
E R W G L O O Y M C Y H C B W T U B E E X G W I O O I M T V
A J I B E P T U F R F O H R F N D T H U B K B S K P M K G F
S Y P N H M O V L I H U E V G M S M B E C O U Y U C B Q L F
U A G I I I R I J W I H V T D A T Q U P E R Q P V W H X E J
E U R L C H E O S E R M R E T Z V S K I C L K R A Q K Y E S
J I A X O U C V C Y M W E P Q R B P Q E R L S K C T O Z H E
D E I G C O E X K J C A N C N G A W Z Z V B B R D L N O L E
P P S N H R P T U W K F C P C W V T W J R F I L E Y R W P O
E U B P L C T I N I B V I N V N O N C K Y T I L U W H U P Q
Y K G J E N O L Q Q I C T S U T O J E O V Q H Y I G O C O K
U Y B O A W R M O V V H P L R G G O I R P X W O W U C H P P
X M A O G Y F S F V A O O J E H S J M C R W A T Q P Q J K G
Y N R S S P X T E F F X N T E I X N X R L P K C K R R E M A
```

aqueous humor
brain
chemoreceptor
cochlea
equilibrium
eyeball
fovea
glutamate
gustation
incus

iris
lens
optic nerve
photoreceptor
pupil
retina
stereocilia
taste
utricle
vestibule

9 Endocrine Control

LEARNING OBJECTIVES

1. Describe the sources, transport, and functions of hormones and neurohormones.
2. Identify the major endocrine glands, locate them in the body, and describe the hormones secreted by each gland.
3. Describe how endocrine glands are regulated.
4. Compare how protein hormones work through second messengers with how steroid hormones work.
5. Justify the reputation of the hypothalamus as the link between nervous and endocrine systems. (Describe the mechanisms by which the hypothalamus exerts its control.)
6. Compare the functions of the posterior and anterior lobes of the pituitary, and describe the actions of their hormones.
7. Summarize the actions of the thyroid hormones and draw a diagram illustrating how they are regulated.
8. Describe how the parathyroid and thyroid glands regulate calcium concentration.
9. Contrast the actions of insulin and glucagon, and describe the disorder diabetes mellitus.
10. Describe the adrenal medulla's responses to stress.
11. Describe the actions of the hormones secreted by the adrenal cortex: glucocorticoids, mineralocorticoids, and sex hormones.
12. Describe the actions of hormones secreted by the pineal gland, thymus gland, atrium of the heart, digestive tract, and adipose tissue.

PART 1: LEARN THE TERMS

Match the following terms to the correct definitions by writing the corresponding letter in the space provided. (Section I)

A. endocrine gland   B. endocrine system   C. endocrinology   D. exocrine gland
E. hormones   F. neuroendocrine cells   G. neurohormone   H. prostaglandins
I. target cells

1. _____ chemical messengers that help regulate body activities

2. _____ study of the endocrine system

3. _____ neurons that are important links between the nervous and endocrine systems

4. _____ helps regulate growth and reproduction; works with nervous system to maintain homeostasis

5. _____ specific cells on which hormones act

6. _____ release secretions into ducts; sweat glands

7. _____ has no ducts; releases hormones into surrounding interstitial (tissue) fluid or into blood

8. _____ produced by neuroendocrine cells; transported down axons and released into interstitial fluid

9. _____ closely related group of lipids; interact with other hormones to regulate various metabolic activities

Fill in the blanks with the correct answer for each statement. (Section II)

10. _____ depends on normal concentrations of hormones in the blood and tissues.

11. Hormone secretion is regulated by _____ systems, neuroendocrine regulation, and _____.

12. In a negative feedback system, information about the amount of _____ in the blood or interstitial fluid is fed back to the endocrine gland.

13. The calcium concentration of the blood is regulated by the _____ glands.

14. An increase in the calcium concentration results in a _____ in parathyroid hormone release; a decrease in calcium concentration leads to _____ parathyroid hormone secretion.

15. _____ regulation involves action of both the nervous and the endocrine systems.

16. The hypothalamus signals the sympathetic_____ system in response to input from stressors and sensory receptors; sympathetic nerves then signal the adrenal glands to release epinephrine and _____.

17. _____ regulate hormones such as the adrenal hormone cortisol.

18. _____ is secreted in a circadian rhythm with greatest secretion in the morning and then _____ throughout the day until reaching its lowest concentration at bedtime.

19. In _____, a gland decreases its hormone output to abnormally low levels, which deprives target cells of needed stimulation.

20. In _____, a gland increases its output to abnormally high levels, overstimulating target cells.

Match the term on the left to the correct selection on the right. (Section III)

21. _____ G protein
22. _____ receptors
23. _____ cyclic AMP
24. _____ calmodulin
25. _____ second messenger
26. _____ steroid hormones
27. _____ first messenger

A. they activate genes

B. typically needed for activation of protein hormones

C. hormone that turns a system on

D. receptor protein associated with the plasma membrane

E. specialized proteins; some bind with hormone molecules

F. a common second messenger

G. protein that binds calcium ions, and then changes shape and can activate enzymes that regulate certain cell processes

Fill in the blanks with the correct answer for each statement. (Section IV)

28. The hypothalamus regulates the _____ gland and secretes several neurohormones, such as oxytocin and antidiuretic hormone.

29. The hypothalamus also secretes releasing hormones and _____, which regulate secretion of several pituitary hormones.

30. At least seven distinct hormones are secreted by the _____ gland, which controls the activities of several other endocrine glands and influence many _____.

31. The _____ of the pituitary gland secretes oxytocin and _____.

32. _____ stimulates contraction of smooth muscle in the wall of the uterus during childbirth and stimulates release of milk from the breast.

33. Antidiuretic hormone (ADH) regulates fluid balance in the body and indirectly helps control _____; it helps the body conserve water by increasing water reabsorption from collecting ducts in the _____.

34. ADH deficiency can lead to a metabolic disorder called _____, in which enormous quantities of dilute urine may be excreted causing serious dehydration.

35. The _____ of the pituitary gland secretes growth hormone, prolactin, and several _____ that stimulate other endocrine glands.

36. Each anterior pituitary hormone is regulated by a _____, and in some cases also by an inhibiting hormone, produced in the hypothalamus.

37. The neurohormones enter capillaries and pass through special _____ that connect the hypothalamus with the anterior lobe of the pituitary.

38. Portal veins do not deliver blood to a larger vein directly but instead connect two sets of _____; releasing and inhibiting hormones pass through the walls of these capillaries into _____ tissue.

Match the following terms to the correct definitions by writing the corresponding letter in the space provided. (Section IV)

A. acromegaly	B. adrenocorticotropic	C. gigantism	D. gonadotropic	E. growth hormone
F. insulin-like	G. pituitary dwarf	H. prolactin	I. somatomedins	J. thyroid-stimulating

39. _____ stimulates cells of the mammary glands to secrete milk during lactation

40. _____ promote growth of the skeleton and stimulate general tissue growth by promoting protein synthesis

41. _____ tropic hormone that stimulates the thyroid gland

42. _____ condition of abnormally tall person due to excess secretion of GH during childhood

43. _____ tropic hormone that stimulates the adrenal cortex

44. _____ condition resulting from hypersecretion of GH during adulthood; characterized by enlarged extremities and face

45. _____ somatomedin peptide growth factors

46. _____ follicle-stimulating and luteinizing tropic hormones that control gonad activities

47. _____ stimulates body growth mainly by stimulating protein synthesis; somatotropin

48. _____ small person whose pituitary gland did not produce enough GH during childhood

Fill in the blanks with the correct answer for each statement. (Section V)

49. The _____ is located in the neck, lying anterior to the trachea and just below the larynx; it secretes two

    thyroid hormones and a hormone called _____.

50. Thyroid hormones are essential for normal growth and _____; they increase _____ rate in
    most tissues.

51. _____, also known as T_4 (because it has four iodine atoms in its structure), is the main thyroid
    hormone.

52. A second hormone, T_3, called _____, has three iodine atoms in its structure.

53. The regulation of thyroid hormone secretion depends on a _____ feedback system between the

    _____ and the thyroid gland.

54. The anterior pituitary secretes _____, which promotes synthesis and secretion of thyroid hormones;

    more TSH is secreted when the normal concentration of thyroid hormones in the blood _____.

55. Extreme _____ during childhood results in low metabolic rate and retarded mental and physical

    development; the condition is called _____.

56. A _____, an abnormal enlargement of the thyroid gland, may be associated with either hyposecretion

    or _____.

57. A person with iodine deficiency develops a goiter because _____ cannot be made; thyroid hormone

    concentration decreases and the anterior pituitary secretes large amounts of TSH causing the _____ to
    enlarge.

Unscramble each term and match it to its correct description. (Section VI)

58. _____ muccial

59. _____ raprayhodit nalgd

60. _____ ynttea

61. _____ citlincano

62. _____ hipardatyro

A. hormone; small protein that regulates calcium level of blood and tissue fluid

B. hormone that inhibits removal of calcium from bone

C. parathyroid glands are regulated by the concentration of this

D. embedded in connective tissue surrounding thyroid gland

E. muscle spasm condition caused by low calcium level due to low PTH secretion

Fill in the blanks with the correct answer for each statement. (Section VII)

63. The pancreas, located in the _____ posterior to the stomach, contains over 1 million scattered clusters

    of cells called _____.

64. About 70% of the islet cells are beta cells that produce the hormone _____; _____ secrete
    the hormone glucagon.

65. Insulin _____ the concentration of glucose in the blood and stimulates cells of many tissues (including
    liver and muscle) to take up glucose from the blood.

66. Glucagon _____ the blood glucose level by stimulating liver cells to convert glycogen to glucose.

67. Insulin and glucagon work _____, using negative feedback, to keep blood glucose concentration within
    normal limits.

68. _____ is the main disorder associated with pancreatic hormones.

69. Insulin-dependent diabetes, referred to as _____, is an autoimmune disorder in which cells of the _____ (misguided T lymphocytes) kill the body's own beta cells.

70. Type 1 diabetes is clinically treated with _____ or the use of an insulin pump.

71. About 90% of all cases of diabetes are non-insulin-dependent, or _____.

72. A common first sign of type 2 diabetes is _____; insulin receptors on _____ cells are not able to bind with insulin and use it.

73. Glucose levels in the blood rise because cells cannot take up _____; blood glucose concentration can become so high that glucose is excreted in the _____.

Match the term on the left to the correct selection on the right. (Section VII)

74. _____ adrenal glands

75. _____ sex hormones

76. _____ androgens

77. _____ mineralocorticoids

78. _____ cortisol

79. _____ adrenal cortex

80. _____ adrenal medulla

81. _____ glucocorticoids

82. _____ aldosterone

83. _____ estrogens

A. main glucocorticoid; also called hydrocortisone

B. secretes three different types of steroid hormones

C. paired glands; small yellow masses of tissue located above the kidneys

D. adrenal cortex secretes these in both sexes

E. emergency gland of body; secretes epinephrine and norepinephrine

F. help body cope with stress; promote glucose production; reduce inflammation

G. principal mineralocorticoid; maintains homeostasis of sodium and potassium ions

H. help regulate water and salt balance

I. female sex hormones

J. hormones that have masculinizing effects

Fill in the blanks with the correct answer for each statement. (Section VII)

84. Stress stimulates the hypothalamus to secrete _____, which stimulates the anterior pituitary to secrete ACTH (adrenocorticotropic hormone);

85. ACTH regulates both _____ and _____ secretion.

86. Abnormally large amounts of glucocorticoids can result in _____ in which fat moves from the lower part of the body and is deposited about the trunk; blood glucose concentration rises up to 50% above normal, causing _____.

87. Hyposecretion of cortisol by the adrenal cortex can lead to _____; the body cannot effectively regulate the concentration of _____ in the blood and the patient loses the ability to cope with stress.

88. _____ may threaten homeostasis, putting the body in a state of stress.

89. When stressed, the brain sends messages activating the _____ and the adrenal glands.

90. Epinephrine and _____ are released, and the body prepares for fight or flight; the hypothalamus signals the _____ to secrete ACTH, increasing cortisol secretion.

91. Chronic _____, which may last for weeks or even years, is harmful because of the effects of long-term elevation of some hormones.

92. The _____ produces melatonin, which regulates biological rhythms, the onset of sexual maturity, and facilitates the onset of sleep.

93. Thymosin, a hormone produced by the _____, plays an important role in immune responses by stimulating proliferation of T cells (T lymphocytes) during infection.

94. The digestive tract and _____ secrete hormones that regulate digestive processes, appetite, and energy metabolism.

95. The atrium of the heart secretes _____, which promotes sodium excretion and lowers _____.

96. Label the endocrine glands in Figure 9-1.

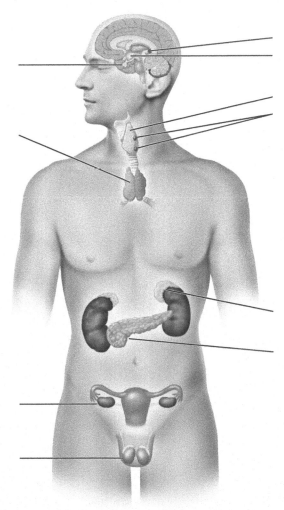

Figure 9-1

Select the correct answer.

1. The endocrine system works with the nervous system to maintain homeostasis by helping to regulate
   a. growth
   b. response to stress
   c. reproduction
   d. all of the above

2. Endocrine glands secrete hormones into surrounding interstitial (tissue) fluid or into the blood to act on

   _____ cells.
   a. target
   b. connective
   c. helper
   d. action

3. Prostaglandins have the following functions:
   a. raise blood pressure
   b. reduce blood pressure
   c. increase secretions in the stomach
   d. both a and b

4. The _____ glands regulate the calcium

   concentration of the blood by _____
   a. adrenal; negative feedback systems
   b. parathyroid; positive feedback systems
   c. parathyroid; negative feedback systems
   d. adrenal; positive feedback systems

5. Which of the following does *not* regulate secretion of hormones
   a. positive feedback systems
   b. negative feedback systems
   c. biological rhythms
   d. neuroendocrine regulation

6. The adrenal hormone _____ is secreted in a circadian rhythm that follows the 24-hour day sleep-wake cycle.
   a. oxytocin
   b. cortisol
   c. somatropin
   d. G protein

7. In _____, a gland increases its output to abnormally high levels, overstimulating the

   _____, which can lead to loss of homeostasis.
   a. hyposecretion; target cells
   b. hypersecretion; target cells
   c. hypersecretion; lymph system
   d. hypersecretion; brain

8. When a protein hormone combines with

   _____ on the plasma membrane of the target cell, information is relayed to a

   _____
   a. receptors; first messenger
   b. enzymes; second messenger
   c. receptors; second messenger
   d. calcium; second messenger

9. The hypothalamus does all of the following *except*
   a. regulates most endocrine activity
   b. secretes thyroxine
   c. regulates the pituitary gland
   d. produces oxytocin

10. The _____ gland, consisting of two main lobes, controls the activities of several other endocrine glands and influences many body processes.
    a. parathyroid
    b. thyroid
    c. pituitary
    d. adrenal

11. Which of the following is a function of oxytocin?
    a. stimulates uterine contractions in childbirth
    b. stimulates body growth by stimulating protein synthesis
    c. facilitates attachment (bonding) between a mother and infant
    d. both a and c

12. Antidiuretic hormone (ADH) regulates

    _____ in the body.
    a. fluid balance
    b. glucose
    c. lactation (milk production)
    d. protein synthesis

13. The anterior lobe of the pituitary gland secretes all of the following *except*
    a. prolactin
    b. adrenocorticotropic hormone
    c. growth hormone
    d. oxytocin

87

14. The _____ regulate(s) the activities of the gonads (ovaries and testes).
    a. adrenocorticotropic hormone (ACTH)
    b. thyroid-stimulating hormone (TSH)
    c. gonadotropic hormones
    d. somatomedins

15. Growth hormone (GH, also called somatotropin) stimulates body growth mainly by stimulating

    _____
    a. luteinizing hormone secretion
    b. metabolism
    c. protein synthesis
    d. muscle cells

Mark each statement true or false; correct the false statements to make them true.

16. _____ The regulation of thyroid hormone secretion depends on a positive feedback system between the posterior pituitary and the thyroid gland.

17. _____ Abnormal enlargement of the thyroid gland is termed a goiter and may be associated with cretinism.

18. _____ When the calcium concentration rises above normal, the parathyroid glands slow their secretion of parathyroid hormone (PTH).

19. _____ Insulin lowers the concentration of glucose in the blood; it stimulates cells of the liver, muscle, and fat to take up glucose from the blood.

20. _____ Glucagon lowers the blood glucose level by stimulating liver cells to convert glycogen to glucose.

21. _____ Type 1 diabetes is an autoimmune disorder in which certain misguided T lymphocytes kill the body's own beta cells resulting in insulin deficiency.

22. _____ The adrenal medulla develops from nervous tissue and its hormone release is controlled by the parasympathetic nervous system.

23. _____ When the body is not under stress, high levels of cortisol in the blood inhibit both CRF (corticotropin-releasing factor) secretion by the hypothalamus and ACTH (adrenocorticotropic hormone) secretion by the pituitary.

24. _____ When under stress, the brain sends messages activating the sympathetic nervous system and the adrenal glands; epinephrine and norepinephrine are released, and the body prepares for fight or flight.

25. _____ The thymus gland, located in the brain, produces melatonin, which regulates biological rhythms and facilitates the onset of sleep.

1. Why is it advantageous for endocrine glands to be ductless, releasing their secretions directly into surrounding interstitial (tissue) fluid or into the blood?

2. Why does oxytocin stimulate uterine contraction at the onset of childbirth and not contraction of other smooth muscles, such as the stomach and the intestine?

3. How might a person be affected if continuously exposed to bright light during sleep hours?

Answer the questions to complete the crossword puzzle.

Hormone Happy

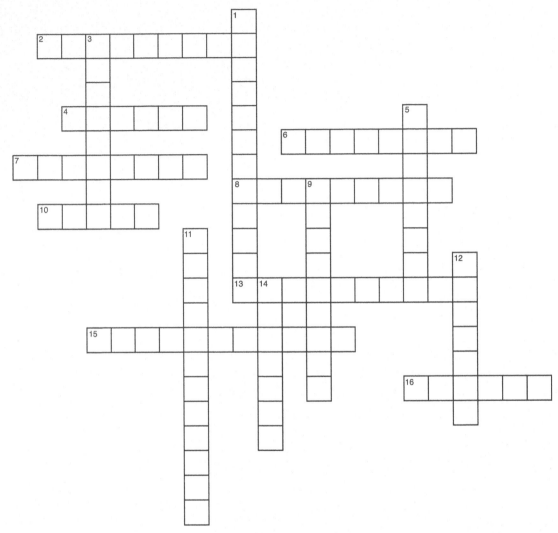

Across

2. stimulates cells of the mammary glands to secrete milk
4. part of heart that secretes hormones
6. secreted in a circadian rhythm
7. organ with islets of Langerhans
8. hormones combine with them on target cells
10. steroid hormones activate them
13. glands that regulate calcium concentration
15. hormone that inhibits removal of calcium from bone
16. abnormal enlargement of the thyroid gland

Down

1. hormone that regulates fluid balance in the body
3. stimulates uterine contraction
5. female sex hormone
9. glands with no ducts
11. regulates pituitary gland
12. lowers the concentration of glucose in the blood
14. glands that function in metabolism and stress

10 The Circulatory System: Blood

CHAPTER GUIDE

I.   The circulatory system performs critical functions
II. Plasma is the fluid component of blood
III. Red blood cells transport oxygen
IV. White blood cells defend the body against disease
V.   Platelets function in blood clotting

VI. Blood must be matched for transfusions
   A. The ABO blood groups are based on antigens A and B
   B. The Rh system consists of several Rh antigens

LEARNING OBJECTIVES

1. List the functions of the circulatory system and describe the composition of blood.
2. Describe the composition of blood plasma and the functions of plasma proteins.
3. Describe the structure, function, and life cycle of red blood cells.
4. Compare the structure and functions of the main types of white blood cells.
5. Describe the structure and function of platelets, and summarize the chemical events in blood clotting.
6. Identify the antigen and antibody associated with each ABO blood type, and explain why blood types must be matched in transfusion therapy.
7. Identify the cause and importance of Rh incompatibility.

PART 1: LEARN THE TERMS

Match the following terms to the correct definitions by writing the corresponding letter in the space provided. (Sections I, II)

A. blood	B. capillaries	C. cardiovascular	D. circulatory	E. heart
F. interstitial fluid	G. intracellular	H. lymphatic	I. plasma	J. plasma proteins

1. _____ pumps blood through the blood vessels

2. _____ pale, yellowish fluid that suspends blood cells and platelets

3. _____ transportation system of the body

4. _____ subsystem that consists of the heart, blood, and blood vessels

5. _____ fluid inside of cells

6. _____ tiniest blood vessels

7. _____ consists of red blood cells, white blood cells, and platelets suspended in plasma

8. _____ three groups contained in plasma with specific properties and functions

9. _____ system helps maintain fluid balance and protects the body against disease

10. _____ tissue fluid that bathes cells

91

Fill in the blanks with the correct answer for each statement. (Section II)

11. Changes in the composition of plasma initiate responses by one or more organs of the body to restore

    _____.

12. Plasma proteins are divided into three groups, or fractions, each with specific _____: (1) albumins,

    (2) globulins, and (3) _____.

13. Plasma proteins, especially _____ and globulins, help regulate the distribution of fluid between

    _____ and interstitial fluid.

14. Plasma proteins (along with hemoglobin in red blood cells) are _____ that help keep the pH of the
    blood within a narrow homeostatic range.

15. Alpha globulins include hormones and proteins that transport hormones; other globulins are _____,
    a protein involved in blood clotting and high-density lipoproteins (HDL), which transport fats

    and _____.

16. _____ include other lipoproteins that transport fats and cholesterol, including low-density lipoproteins

    (LDL), and proteins that transport certain _____ and minerals.

17. The gamma globulin fraction contains _____ that provide immunity to diseases, such as measles and
    infectious hepatitis.

18. _____ and several other plasma proteins are involved in the clotting process; when clotting proteins are

    removed from plasma, the remaining liquid is called _____.

Match the term on the left to the correct selection on the right. (Section III)

19. _____ hemoglobin

20. _____ stem cells

21. _____ oxyhemoglobin

22. _____ anemia

23. _____ red bone marrow

24. _____ iron

25. _____ biconcave

26. _____ hemolytic anemias

27. _____ erythropoietin

28. _____ erythrocytes

A. oxygen combines weakly with hemoglobin to form this

B. thinner in the center than around the edge

C. hormone that regulates red blood cell production

D. anemic condition in which red blood cells are destroyed

E. red blood cells (RBCs); transport oxygen and carbon dioxide; produce
   and package hemoglobin

F. RBCs are produced here

G. red pigment that transports oxygen

H. condition in which there is deficiency in red blood cells and hemoglobin

I. essential ingredient of hemoglobin

J. immature cells that multiply and give rise to blood cells

Fill in the blanks with the correct answer for each statement. (Section IV)

29. White blood cells (WBCs), or _____, are specialized to defend the body against viruses, harmful

    bacteria, and many _____ that cause disease.

30. Although RBCs function within the _____, many WBCs leave the circulation and move through tissues destroying bacteria and engulfing dead cells and foreign matter by the process of _____.

31. Neutrophils, the main _____ in the blood, ingest bacteria and dead cells; granules in neutrophils contain _____ that digest ingested material.

32. Eosinophils have _____ containing enzymes that destroy viruses and bacteria; some of their enzymes kill parasitic _____.

33. _____ have granules in their cytoplasm, which contain histamine, a substance that dilates blood vessels and makes capillaries more permeable; basophils release _____ in injured tissues and in allergic responses.

34. Other basophil granules contain the anticoagulant _____, which helps prevent blood from clotting inappropriately within blood vessels.

35. Some agranular leukocytes are lymphocytes that are specialized to produce _____; other lymphocytes directly attack bacteria and cells that contain viruses.

36. A second type of agranular leukocyte, _____, migrate into connective tissues and develop into macrophages, the large scavenger cells of the body.

37. Monocytes also give rise to _____ cells, which destroy viruses.

38. _____ is a blood cancer in which certain stem cells multiply wildly within the bone marrow, crowding out other types of developing WBCs (and RBCs and platelets); anemia, impaired blood clotting, and _____ result.

Match the following terms to the correct definitions by writing the corresponding letter in the space provided. (Section V)

| A. clotting factors | B. fibrin | C. fibrinogen | D. liver |
| E. platelet plug | F. prothrombin activator | G. thrombin | H. thrombocytes |

39. _____ catalyzes the conversion of prothrombin to its active form

40. _____ platelets; tiny fragments of cytoplasm that prevent blood loss

41. _____ platelets and injured tissue release substances that activate these

42. _____ acts as an enzyme that converts the plasma protein fibrinogen to fibrin

43. _____ seals holes in the blood vessel wall

44. _____ prothrombin is manufactured in this organ

45. _____ protein that forms long threads; the webbing of the clot

46. _____ plasma protein that is converted to fibrin

Fill in the blanks with the correct answer for each statement. (Section VI)

47. A blood _____, the transfer of whole blood, plasma, platelets, or other blood components from a healthy donor to a _____ is a routine, lifesaving procedure.

48. Blood components are _____ at high speed to separate the blood so that the heavier components settle at the bottom of a tube.

49. Donor and recipient blood must be carefully _____ for compatibility before transfusion to prevent a transfusion reaction.

50. A transfusion reaction is a serious allergic reaction in which _____ in the recipient's blood attack the foreign red blood cells in the transfused blood, causing them to _____, or clump.

51. In the process of _____ red blood cells rupture, releasing hemoglobin into the plasma.

52. Red blood cells present specific proteins, called _____, on their surfaces, which are different in persons with different blood types.

53. _____, found in the plasma, are specific proteins that recognize and bind to specific antigens.

54. Persons with type A blood have _____ antibodies circulating in their blood and can safely receive only A type blood; those with type B blood have _____ antibodies and must be transfused with type B blood.

55. Persons with _____ blood have neither type of antibody; they are referred to as _____ because they can be transfused with any type blood.

56. Individuals with _____ blood have both types of antibodies; they are called _____ because their blood can be safely used by people of all blood types.

57. An Rh antigen is referred to as an _____; the most important of the many Rh factors is

_____.

58. Most persons of Western European descent have antigen D on the surfaces of their red blood cells and are said to be _____; about 5% of the population who are Rh-negative have no _____ on their RBC surfaces.

59. Antibody D does not occur in the blood of _____ persons unless they have been exposed to antigen D.

60. Rh _____ occurs in a fetus or newborn when the mother's Rh-positive antibodies cross the _____ and causes hemolysis of the baby's red blood cells.

PART 2: ASSESS YOUR UNDERSTANDING

Select the correct answer.

1. The circulatory system, or transportation system, of the body consists of two subsystems, the

_____ system and the _____ system.
   a. nervous; lymphatic
   b. cardiovascular; respiratory
   c. cardiovascular; lymphatic
   d. nervous; respiratory

2. Which of the following is transported by the blood?
   a. nutrients
   b. oxygen and carbon dioxide
   c. hormones
   d. all of the above

3. The cardiovascular system does all of the following *except*
   a. secretes a hormone that helps regulate the posterior pituitary gland
   b. helps regulate acid-base balance
   c. protects the body against disease-causing organisms
   d. transports nutrients from the digestive system to all of the cells

4. Blood consists of
   a. red blood cells, plasma cells, and white blood cells
   b. red blood cells, white blood cells, and endocrine cells
   c. plasma cells, red blood cells, and platelets
   d. red blood cells, white blood cells, platelets, and plasma

5. Substances continuously move into and out of the _____ as blood passes through the _____.
   a. circulation; heart
   b. plasma; capillaries
   c. liver; heart
   d. red blood cells; veins

6. Which of the following is *not* a plasma protein, or fraction?
   a. albumin
   b. fibrogen
   c. glycogen
   d. globulins

7. Beta globulins include
   a. lipoproteins that transport fats and cholesterol
   b. low-density lipoproteins (LDL)
   c. proteins that transport some vitamins and minerals
   d. all of the above

8. The _____ fraction contains antibodies that provide immunity to diseases, such as measles and infectious hepatitis.
   a. alpha globulin
   b. beta globulin
   c. gamma globulin
   d. none of the above

9. Which of the following is *not* a characteristic of red blood cells?
   a. have large nucleus
   b. transport oxygen and carbon dioxide
   c. produce and package hemoglobin
   d. are biconcave

10. Red blood cell production is regulated by the hormone _____, which is secreted by the _____ in response to decreased oxygen concentration.
    a. thrombin; liver
    b. erythropoietin; liver
    c. erythropoietin; kidneys
    d. thrombin; kidneys

11. White blood cells develop from stem cells in the _____ and some leave the _____ to protect the body against pathogens.
    a. red bone marrow; circulation
    b. kidneys; body
    c. yellow bone marrow; circulation
    d. red bone marrow; body

12. _____ are the main phagocytes in the blood seeking out and ingesting bacteria and phagocytizing dead cells.
    a. basophils
    b. neutrophils
    c. eosinophils
    d. red blood cells

13. _____ release histamine in injured tissues and in allergic responses and also release heparin, an anticoagulant that helps prevent blood from clotting.
    a. neutrophils
    b. eosinophils
    c. platelets
    d. basophils

14. Which of the following is *not* true of eosinophils?
    a. contain enzymes that are especially toxic to parasitic worms
    b. phagocytize bacteria and dead cells
    c. play an important role in allergic reactions
    d. have numerous granules that stain red

Mark each statement true or false; correct the false statements to make them true.

15. _____ Monocytes migrate into connective tissues and develop into macrophages; monocytes also give rise to dendritic cells, which destroy viruses.

16. _____ Platelets are cells that prevent blood loss by forming a platelet plug that seals the hole in a blood vessel wall.

17. _____ The blood of a donor and recipient must be carefully matched because a transfusion reaction can occur if their blood is not compatible.

18. _____ Individuals with type AB blood have neither type of antigen on their RBCs and are referred to as universal donors.

19. _____ Individuals with type AB blood have antibodies to both type A or type B blood and can safely receive blood of any ABO type.

20. _____ When an Rh-negative woman and an Rh-positive man produce an Rh-positive baby, the mother may be exposed to antigen D.

PART 3: ACCEPT THE CHALLENGE

1. If an individual allergic to nuts is exposed to peanut butter, which leukocytes are likely to play a major role in the ensuing allergic response?

2. What would be the effect of platelet transfusion between individuals with different ABO blood types?

3. If an Rh-negative woman has several Rh-positive children, will Rh incompatibility continue to be a problem with each additional child?

THE PUZZLE

Find and circle the following words from Chapter 10. Words may be found from top to bottom, bottom to top, right to left, left to right, and diagonally.

```
O C G R A N U L A R S I Q M J J O G Y R L C J T F E M N A Q
B I A B A E S V F Q G E V N I K O B U B N Z V S C K N G S N
L U A Q R U Q N Y U O T Y K L W I N C Y O L S L L B D V I Y
H U V Q I C A Y L P H Y Y A V I M L B F I Q X K O Z O Y U R
D A H H M F O M T S J C N D B D H C Q L K P M E T I A B H B
L S M G U U M J U H L O K I G D D P W R L L I V T Q G G Z R
Q V U S P I K M Y Q Q K C T G T M A O Z K Y L P I D O K S T
C X J N A C L O Y M T U A O L E O O O R G J X H N N A M S A
A V A T F L W X M K E E G U U J F K U R T A K A G W T D R J
F Y A I L D P R E Y V L B Q J C D R E D K U D L C L B Y X M
N I N E T Y C O N O M H I W B O W N Q R H G E F I C N N H Q
I L B T R R T V V Y X P C O G L J H T S C E Y N R B Y D Y J
G O O R G V I U C H E H O Z R E U Z X V H E P B C U R Z L E
Q E A X I S J S S G O I N T A F U A E T A N I T U L G G A O
J T M E A N V Z L R S Q C V B P Q N E U N D P I L Y Y P U L
I Y L D U P O K X W I P A F P O X O M N J H G K A U I A O W
R C I T X U C G G C N O V N M G A Z C T V F C E T P N Q G G
M O L Q J J Y A H E V O K E C Z C I W D X Q G P Q O K I M Y U
Z H M X P Q N N K N P I T J C I M W K R Q T G H R Z B I W P
L P M Y R T T I N F H N L O K A E A P V G Z M J J Y W O Z O Y
U M U S X K I N N F I G T O D V N A M G T G E P Y C L D R M
F Y D J Y E G H K Z L X B Y O U A Z G F L U M T S Z G U A A
T L K Q D X E T O Y N B B E B A A M C Z S O X Z I R O Z O M
P A D S B J N W H D A L Q H M I H E O Q J Y B N I Z M M S S
S O W N P G V K P N I B M O R H T O R P H L L U W X E X H R
X V D F M Y A Y I L D Y Q S Q W K Q B I N C O R L D H O G N
Z V I B K J R N V L B U X E G A H P O R C A M W L I L D R T
J O P W T V H A R D E G W C L S P O Z K Y Y T K N V N X L B
M D W J M J W H K Y A S O E G M L V H C D Q M J Q R R Y N Y
L L I H P O S A B D W N J C H J M G P H A G O C Y T O S I S
```

agglutinate
anemia
antigen
basophil
biconcave
circulatory
clotting
eosinophil
fibrinogen
globulin

granular
hemoglobin
leukocyte
lymphocyte
macrophage
monocyte
neutrophil
phagocytosis
plasma
prothrombin

11 The Circulatory System: The Heart

CHAPTER GUIDE

I.   The heart wall consists of three layers
II. The heart has four chambers
III. Valves prevent backflow of blood
IV. The heart has its own blood vessels
V.   The conduction system consists of specialized cardiac muscle

VI.   The cardiac cycle includes contraction and relaxation phases
VII. Cardiac output depends on stroke volume and heart rate
VIII. The heart is regulated by the nervous and endocrine systems

LEARNING OBJECTIVES

1. Locate the heart and describe the structure of its wall.
2. Identify the chambers of the heart and compare their functions.
3. Locate the atrioventricular and semilunar valves and compare their functions.
4. Identify the principal blood vessels that serve the heart wall.

5. Trace the path of an electrical impulse through the conduction system of the heart.
6. Describe the events of the cardiac cycle and correlate them with normal heart sounds.
7. Define cardiac output and identify factors that affect it.
8. Describe how the nervous and endocrine systems regulate the heart.

PART 1: LEARN THE TERMS

Match the following terms to the correct definitions by writing the corresponding letter in the space provided. (Section I)

A. endocarium
B. endothelium
C. epicardium
D. heart
E. myocardium
F. parietal pericardium
G. pericardial cavity
H. pericardium

1. _____ muscular organ located in thorax between the lungs; pumps blood throughout the body

2. _____ outer layer of the heart; also called visceral pericardium; inner layer of pericardium

3. _____ innermost layer of the heart; consists of smooth endothelial lining resting on connective tissue

4. _____ outer layer of pericardium; strong sac that helps to anchor heart within the thorax

5. _____ space between two layers of pericardium

6. _____ smooth lining of the endocardium consisting of endothelial cells

7. _____ two-layer sac enclosing the heart

8. _____ middle layer of the heart wall; cardiac muscle that contracts to pump the blood

Fill in the blanks with the correct answer for each statement. (Sections 1, II)

9. The heart is a hollow, fist-sized, muscular _____ that can pump from 5 to 35 liters of _____ per minute, depending on the body's needs.

10. The wall of the heart is richly supplied with nerves, blood vessels, and _____.

11. The heart is a double pump with the right and left sides completely separated by a wall, or _____.

12. The atria receive blood _____ to the heart from the veins and act as _____ between contractions of the heart.

13. The _____ pump blood into the great arteries _____ the heart.

14. The _____ receives oxygen-poor blood returning from the tissues, and the right ventricle pumps it into the _____ circulation, the system of blood vessels that connect the heart and lungs.

15. Pulmonary arteries carry blood to the _____, where gases are exchanged; pulmonary _____ then return oxygen-rich blood to the left atrium.

16. The _____ pumps oxygen-rich blood into the aorta, the largest artery of the _____ circulation; this network of blood vessels then delivers blood to all of the body systems.

17. The _____ is the wall between the atria; the wall between the _____ is the interventricular septum.

18. A small, muscular pouch called the _____ increases the surface area of each atrium.

Match the term on the left to the correct selection on the right. (Section III)

19. _____ cusps

20. _____ tricuspid

21. _____ semilunar

22. _____ pulmonary semilunar

23. _____ atrioventricular (AV)

24. _____ chordae tendineae

25. _____ bicuspid

26. _____ aortic semilunar

A. connective tissue cords that hold AV valves in place; heart strings

B. valves that guard the passageway between each atrium and ventricle; prevent blood backflow

C. valve between the left ventricle and the aorta

D. flaps of fibrous tissues that project from the heart wall; part of the AV valve

E. left AV valve, which has two cusps; mitral valve

F. valves that guard the exits from the ventricles

G. AV valve between the right atrium and the right ventricle, which has three cusps

H. valve between the right ventricle and the pulmonary artery

Unscramble each term and match it to its correct description. (Section IV)

27. _____ nayorcor tayrer isdeeas

28. _____ ncoryoar tesarrie

29. _____ oymlacdrai rnictaonfi

30. _____ ocnroyar sivne

31. _____ yrrnaoco nussi

32. _____ ciimhesc

A. empties into the right atrium

B. these vessels join to form the coronary sinus

C. lacking in blood supply

D. branches of these two vessels bring blood to all heart tissue

E. develops when coronary arteries or their branches become thickened or blocked, reducing blood flow

F. cardiac tissue is deprived of adequate supply of oxygen and nutrients leading to this

Fill in the blanks with the correct answer for each statement. (Section V)

33. The heart can beat independently of its nerve supply because it has its own specialized _____, which includes the sinoatrial node, the _____ node, and the atrioventricular bundle.

34. Each heartbeat is initiated by the _____ node, or pacemaker, which is a small mass of specialized muscle in the posterior wall of the _____.

35. One group of atrial muscle fibers conducts the _____ directly to the AV node, located in the right atrium along the lower part of the septum.

36. Transmission of the impulse is delayed briefly to allow the _____ to complete their contraction before the _____ begin to contract.

37. The impulse spreads from the AV node into specialized _____ that form the AV bundle.

38. The AV bundle splits and extends into the right and left _____ where fibers of the bundle branches divide into smaller branches ending in terminal fibers known as _____.

39. The Purkinje fibers extend from fibers of ordinary cardiac muscle within the _____, and the impulse spreads through the ventricles.

40. Cardiac muscle fibers are joined at their ends by dense bands called _____, tight junctions between the muscle cells that allow _____ to pass rapidly from cell to cell.

Fill in the blanks to correctly complete each sentence, and then unscramble the circled letters to correctly complete the final sentence. (Section VI)

41. A _ _ _ ◯ _ _ _ cycle consists of a contraction in which blood is forced out of the heart and then a relaxation in which the heart fills with blood.

42. The period of contraction is called systole; the period of relaxation is _ ◯ _ _ _ _ _ ◯.

43. A cardiac cycle begins with an electrical impulse that spreads from the sinoatrial (SA) node throughout the atria, resulting in the _ ◯ _ _ _ _ _ _ _ _ _ of the atria.

44. When the atria contract, they force blood through the open _ _ _ _ _ _ _ ◯ into the ventricles; the semilunar valves are closed during this part of the cardiac cycle.

45. As the atria relax, they are filled with blood from the veins; during this time, the AV valves are closed and the ventricles are contracting, forcing blood through the ◯ _ _ _ _ _ _ _ ◯ valves into the arteries.

46. As the ventricles begin to ◯ _ _ _ _ _, the semilunar valves close and the AV valves open; blood flows into the ventricles, and the cycle begins again.

47. The electrical activity of the heart can be _ _ _ _ _ _ _ _ ◯ and recorded by an electrocardiograph; the written record, called an electrocardiogram (ECG), can document abnormalities, which may indicate heart disorders.

48. Heart murmurs are abnormal heart sounds that may indicate valve _ _ _ _ _ _ _ _ _ _; when a valve does not close properly, some blood may flow backward resulting in a hissing sound.

Match the following terms to the correct definitions by writing the corresponding letter in the space provided. (Sections VII, VIII)

A. acetylcholine	**B. bradycardia**	**C. cardiac centers**	**D. cardiac output**	**E. heart rate**
F. norepinephrine	**G. Starling's law**	**H. stroke volume**	**I. tachycardia**	**J. venous return**

49. _____ amount of blood delivered to the heart by the veins

50. _____ volume of blood pumped by the left ventricle into the aorta in 1 minute

51. _____ number of ventricular contractions per minute

52. _____ slow heart rate; less than 60 beats per minute

53. _____ in medulla of the brain; maintain control over parasympathetic and sympathetic nerves, which signal the SA node

54. _____ volume of blood pumped by one ventricle during one beat

55. _____ fast heart rate; more than 100 beats per minute

56. _____ the more blood delivered to the heart by the veins, the more blood the heart pumps

57. _____ parasympathetic nerves release this neurotransmitter, which slows the heart

58. _____ sympathetic nerves release this, which speeds heart rate and increases strength of contraction

59. Label the parts of the heart in Figure 11-1.

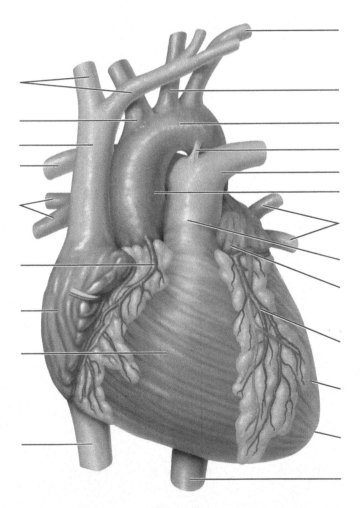

Figure 11-1

60. Label the parts of the heart in Figure 11-2.

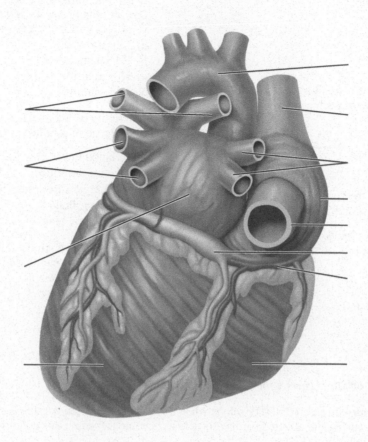

Figure 11-2

PART 2: ASSESS YOUR UNDERSTANDING

Select the correct answer.

1. Which of the following is *not* correct concerning the heart?
   a. it has four chambers
   b. the heart wall consists of three layers
   c. it is located in the abdomen
   d. it has its own blood vessels

2. From the inside out, the layers of the heart are the
   a. endocardium, myocardium, and pericardium
   b. pericardium, endothelium, and myocardium
   c. pericardium, myocardium, and endocardium
   d. myocardium, endothelium, and pericardium

3. The greatest bulk of the heart wall is the

   _____, the cardiac muscle that contracts to pump the blood.
   a. epicardium
   b. myocardium
   c. pericardium
   d. epithelium

4. The two layers of the pericardium are the
   a. epicardium and myocardium
   b. epicardium and parietal pericardium
   c. epithelium and parietal pericardium
   d. myocardium and endocardium

5. The right atrium receives oxygen-poor blood (blood somewhat depleted of its oxygen supply) returning from the tissues, and the right ventricle pumps it into the
   a. right ventricle
   b. left ventricle
   c. pulmonary circulation
   d. left atrium

6. Pulmonary veins return oxygen-rich blood to the
   a. right ventricle
   b. left ventricle
   c. left atrium
   d. lungs

7. The systemic circulation, or blood delivery system of the body, begins with the
   a. pulmonary artery
   b. pulmonary vein
   c. aorta
   d. right ventricle

8. The _____ is a small muscular pouch that increases the surface are of each atrium.
   a. aorta
   b. interatrial septum
   c. interventricular septum
   d. auricle

9. The AV valve between the right atrium and the right ventricle has three cusps and is called the

   _____ valve; the AV valve between the left atrium and left ventricle, with two cusps, is the

   _____ valve.
   a. tricuspid; bicuspid
   b. pulmonary; semilunar
   c. bicuspid; tricuspid
   d. semilunar; bicuspid

10. _____ is a common valve deformity in which the mitral valve is thickened and slows the flow of blood from the left atrium into the left ventricle causing the heart to work harder.
    a. Mitral stenosis
    b. Rheumatic fever
    c. Hypertension
    d. Endocarditis

11. The right and left _____ arteries branch from the aorta as it leaves the heart; their branches

    bring blood to the _____.
    a. carotid; lower body
    b. coronary; heart tissue
    c. coronary; brain
    d. pulmonary; brain

12. Blood flows through the _____ after passing through capillaries in the heart wall.
    a. carotid arteries
    b. pulmonary veins
    c. coronary veins
    d. aorta

Mark each statement true or false; correct the false statements to make them true.

13. _____ Coronary artery disease (CAD) develops when thickened or blocked coronary arteries deliver insufficient blood flow causing the affected cardiac muscle to become ischemic; this condition can lead to a myocardial infarction (MI).

14. _____ It is possible for the heart to beat for many hours independently of the rest of the body because the heart has its own specialized conduction system independent of its nerve supply.

15. _____ Each heartbeat is initiated by the AV node, which generates electrical impulses (action potentials) 70 to 80 times each minute.

16. _____ From the AV node the impulse spreads into specialized muscle fibers that form the AV bundle; these large fibers conduct impulses about six times faster than ordinary cardiac muscle fibers.

17. _____ Fibers of the AV bundle branches divide into smaller branches ending in intercalated disks, which extend from fibers of ordinary cardiac muscle within the myocardium.

18. _____ The pathway taken by an electrical impulse through the heart is SA node: cardiac muscle of atria (atria contract) and to AV node, AV bundle, right and left bundle branches, Purkinje fibers, ordinary muscle fibers of ventricles, and then the ventricles contract.

19. _____ The cardiac cycle occurs about 72 times per minute and consists of continuous contractions in which blood is forced out of the heart.

20. _____ The period of contraction is called diastole, which begins with an electrical impulse that spreads from the SA node throughout the atria, resulting in the contraction of the atria.

21. _____ The electrical activity of the heart can be amplified and recorded by an electrocardiograph by placing electrodes on the body surface on opposite sides of the heart.

22. _____ By multiplying the stroke volume by the number of times the left ventricle beats per minute, we can compute the cardiac output (the volume of blood pumped by the left ventricle into the aorta in 1 minute).

23. _____ The cardiac centers in the heart wall maintain control over the two sets of autonomic nerves, parasympathetic and sympathetic nerves, which signal the SA node.

24. _____ Parasympathetic nerves release the neurotransmitter acetylcholine, which slows the heart; sympathetic nerves release norepinephrine, which speeds the heart rate and increases the strength of contraction.

PART 3: ACCEPT THE CHALLENGE

1. Some babies are born with a hole in the septum, or septal defect, between the right and left atria or right and left ventricles. How would this defect affect blood flow in the heart?

2. Based on what you have learned about how the SA node works, describe how a mechanical pacemaker would function to assist the heart.

3. Why is it important to cool a patient's heart before heart surgery is performed?

Answer the questions to complete the crossword puzzle.

Your Beating Heart

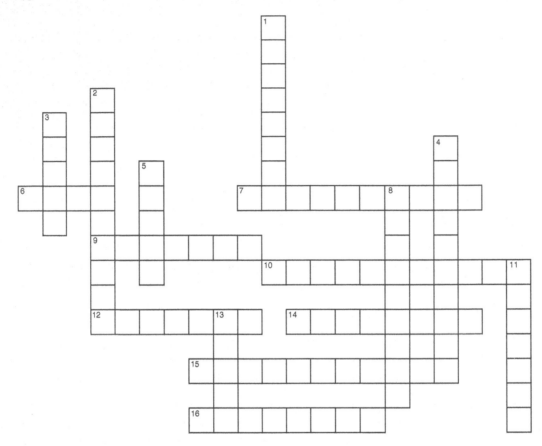

Across

6. number of chambers in the human heart
7. cardiac cycle includes contraction and
9. arteries that supply the heart
10. slow heart rate; less than 60 beats per minute
12. period of contraction
14. mitral valve
15. smooth lining of the endocardium
16. lacking in blood supply

Down

1. period of relaxation
2. muscular chambers below the atria
3. it is pumped throughout the body
4. greatest bulk of the heart wall
5. muscular organ that pumps blood throughout body
8. AV valve between the right atrium and right ventricle
11. increases surface area of each atrium
13. pulmonary artery sends blood here for oxygenation

12 The Circulation of Blood and Lymph

CHAPTER GUIDE

I.   Three main types of blood vessels circulate blood
   A. Arteries carry blood away from the heart
   B. Capillaries are exchange vessels
   C. Veins carry blood back to the heart
II. Blood circulates through two circuits
   A. The pulmonary circulation carries blood to and from the lungs
   B. The systemic circulation carries blood to and from the tissues
     1. The aorta has four main regions
     2. The superior and inferior venae cavae return blood to the heart
     3. Four arteries supply the brain
     4. The liver has an unusual circulation
III. Several factors influence blood flow
   A. The alternate expansion and recoil of an artery is its pulse

   B. Blood pressure depends on blood flow and resistance to blood flow
   C. Pressure changes as blood flows through the systemic circulation
   D. Blood pressure is expressed as systolic pressure over diastolic pressure
   E. Blood pressure must be carefully regulated
IV. The lymphatic system is an accessory circulatory system
   A. The lymph circulation is a drainage system
   B. Lymph nodes filter lymph
   C. Tonsils filter interstitial fluid
   D. The spleen filters blood
   E. The thymus gland plays a role in immune function

LEARNING OBJECTIVES

1. Compare the structure and functions of arteries, capillaries, and veins.
2. Trace a drop of blood through the pulmonary and systemic circulations, listing the principal vessels and heart chambers through which it must pass on its journey from one part of the body to another. (For example, trace a drop of blood from the inferior vena cava to an organ, such as the brain, and then back to the heart.)
3. Identify the main divisions of the aorta and its principal branches.
4. Trace a drop of blood through the brain.
5. Trace a drop of blood through the hepatic portal system.

6. State the physiological basis for arterial pulse and describe how pulse is measured.
7. State the relationship among blood pressure, blood flow, and resistance, and describe how blood pressure is measured.
8. Compare blood pressure in the different types of blood vessels of the systemic circulation.
9. Describe mechanisms by which the nervous and endocrine systems regulate blood pressure.
10. Describe the functions, tissues, and organs of the lymphatic system.
11. Trace the flow of lymph from a lymph capillary to the left or right subclavian vein.

PART 1: LEARN THE TERMS

Match the following terms to the correct definitions by writing the corresponding letter in the space provided. (Section I)

A. arteries   B. arterioles   C. blood vessels   D. capillaries
E. interstitial fluid   F. metarterioles   G. precapillary sphincter   H. sinusoids
I. tunica adventitia   J. tunica media   K. tunica intima   L. veins
M. venules

1. _____ vessels carry blood from ventricles of the heart to organs and tissues of the body

2. _____ nourishes cells and keeps them moist

3. _____ inner layer of an artery or vein wall; consists of endothelium

4. _____ tubes through which blood circulates throughout the body

5. _____ outer layer of an artery or vein wall; consists of connective tissue rich in elastic and collagen fibers

6. _____ thin and somewhat porous blood vessels; some plasma leaks through their walls into tissues

7. _____ smallest veins

8. _____ smallest branches of an artery; important in regulating blood pressure

9. _____ blood vessels that conduct blood back toward the heart

10. _____ middle layer of an artery or vein wall; consists of connective tissue and smooth muscle

11. _____ smooth muscle cell that helps regulate blood supply to each organ and its tissues

12. _____ small vessels that directly link arterioles with venules

13. _____ capillary-like vessels in liver, spleen, and bone marrow that connect arterioles and venules

Fill in the blanks with the correct answer for each statement. (Section II)

14. Blood circulates through two continuous networks of blood vessels: (1) the _____ circulation connects heart and lungs, and (2) the systemic circulation connects the _____ with all of the organs and tissues.

15. The left _____ pumps blood into the _____ circulation, delivering oxygen-rich blood to organs and tissues; oxygen-poor blood loaded with carbon dioxide wastes returns to the right atrium.

16. The right ventricle pumps the blood into the _____ circulation, where gases are exchanged, and the blood is returned to the left _____.

17. Oxygen-poor blood is pumped into the right ventricle and then into the _____, which deliver blood to the lungs.

18. The pulmonary arteries lead to an extensive network of capillaries; as blood flows through the pulmonary capillaries, _____ diffuses out of the blood and oxygen diffuses into it.

19. The _____ return oxygen-rich blood to the left atrium; blood then passes into the left ventricle and is pumped into the systemic circulation again.

20. Blood flows through the pulmonary circulation in the following sequence: right atrium to _____; to pulmonary arteries; then to pulmonary capillaries; to _____ and back to the left atrium.

21. The left ventricle pumps blood into the largest artery, the _____; branches of the aorta deliver blood to all organs and tissues.

22. The first part of the aorta, called the _____, travels upward (superiorly).

23. From the ascending aorta, the _____ curves and makes a U-turn.

24. The thoracic aorta _____ from the aortic arch and passes through the _____, posterior to the heart.

25. The region of the aorta below the diaphragm, the _____, descends downward through the abdominal cavity; the abdominal aorta and thoracic aorta, together, make up the descending aorta.

26. Label the blood vessels and lymphatic vessels in Figure 12-1.

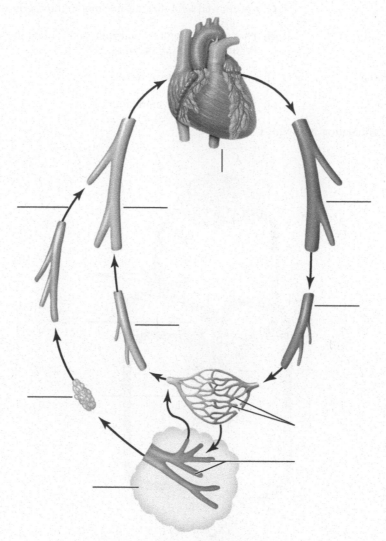

Figure 12-1

Match the term on the left to the correct selection on the right. (Section II)

27. _____ inferior vena cava

28. _____ vertebral arteries

29. _____ internal carotid arteries

30. _____ superior vena cava

31. _____ circle of Willis

32. _____ venous sinus

33. _____ anastomosis

34. _____ basilar artery

35. _____ brachiocephalic

36. _____ internal jugular

A. circle of arteries at the base of the brain

B. receives blood from the upper portions of the body

C. blood circulates through this vein to the superior vena cava

D. receives blood returning from below the level of the diaphragm

E. the two vertebral arteries form this

F. enter cranial cavity in midregion of cranial floor to bring blood to the brain

G. specialized vein that has no smooth muscle in its wall

H. pass through foramen magnum and join on the ventral surface of the brainstem to bring blood to the brain

I. veins at each side of the neck

J. joining of two or more arteries

37. Label the parts of the circulation in Figure 12-2.

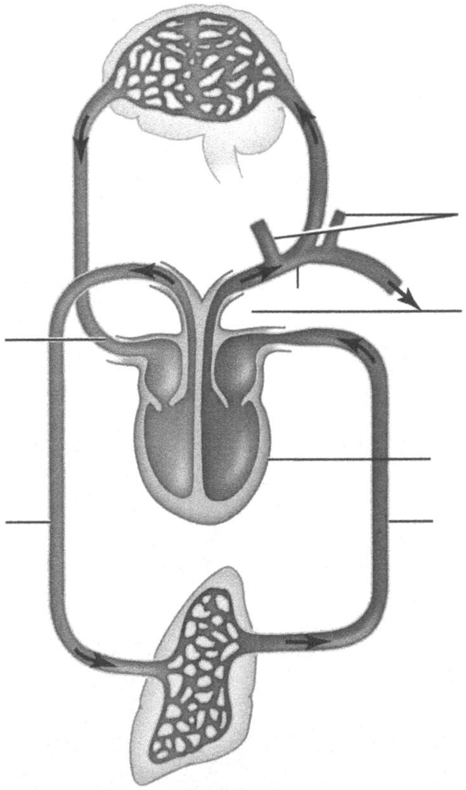

Figure 12-2

Unscramble each term and match it to its correct description. (Section II)

38. opsuerri cirtmesene   A. delivers blood to the intestines

39. ratpol inesv   B. delivers blood from organs of the digestive system to the liver

40. encirmtese eyartr   C. vein that empties into the hepatic portal vein

41. peichat lpator   D. exchange vessels somewhat like capillaries

42. diounisss   E. vein that carries blood to a second set of exchange vessels (capillaries or sinusoids)

Fill in the blank with the correct answer for each statement. (Section III)

43. The elastic wall of the _____ stretches each time the left ventricle pumps blood into the aorta.

44. The alternate arterial expansion and recoil that moves down the aorta and its branches in a wave, faster than the flow of the blood itself, is called the _____.

45. Arterial pulse prevents blood from rushing through arteries and into arterioles and capillaries in enormous gushes each time the _____ contracts; pressure and volume from large gushes would damage the delicate walls of the _____.

46. You can feel your _____ when you place your finger over an artery near the skin surface.

47. Any superficial artery that is located over a bone or other firm structure, such as the common _____ in the neck region, can be used to measure pulse.

48. These locations are referred to as _____ because pressure applied directly on the vessel at these points may stop arterial bleeding if a wound is _____ to the pressure point.

49. The pulse is felt just after the ventricles _____ because it takes time for the pulse wave to pass from the ventricle to the _____.

50. Blood pressure, the force exerted by the _____ against the inner walls of the blood vessels, is determined by the flow of blood and the _____ to that flow.

51. The flow of blood depends directly on the pumping action of the _____; when cardiac output increases, blood flow _____, causing a rise in blood pressure.

52. Blood flow is directly affected by blood _____; if blood volume is reduced by hemorrhage or by chronic bleeding, the blood pressure _____.

53. Peripheral resistance is the opposing force to blood flow caused by _____ of blood and by the friction between blood and the wall of the blood vessel; when peripheral resistance _____, blood pressure increases.

54. The length and _____ of a blood vessel determine the amount of surface area in contact with the blood; a small change in the diameter of a blood vessel (particularly an arteriole) causes a big change in

_____

Match the following terms to the correct definitions by writing the corresponding letter in the space provided. (Section III)

| A. aldosterone | B. angiotensin II | C. baroreceptors | D. blood pressure | E. hypertension |
| F. renin | G. vasoconstriction | H. vasodilation | I. veins | J. vein valves |

55. _____ blood pressure higher than normal; a risk factor for cardiovascular disease

56. _____ prevent backflow that would occur because of the force of gravity

57. _____ kidneys release this enzyme in response to low blood pressure

58. _____ decrease in blood vessel diameter

59. _____ at any time, more than 60% of blood in circulation is found here

60. _____ hormone that signals the kidneys to increase sodium reabsorption

61. _____ specialized receptors in the walls of certain arteries and in the heart wall that are sensitive to changes in blood pressure

62. _____ increase in blood vessel diameter

63. _____ expressed as systolic pressure over diastolic pressure

64. _____ hormone that acts as a powerful vasoconstrictor

Fill in the blank with the correct answer for each statement. (Section IV)

65. The lymphatic system consists of the clear, watery lymph that is formed from _____ fluid, the lymphatic vessels that conduct the lymph, and _____.

66. Lymph tissue is a type of _____ tissue with large numbers of lymphocytes; it is organized into small masses of tissue called _____.

67. The lymph circulation is a _____ system, which collects excess interstitial fluid and returns it to the blood.

68. When interstitial fluid enters dead-ended lymph _____, it is called lymph; lymph capillaries conduct lymph to larger vessels called lymphatics, which enter _____ at strategic locations.

69. Lymph flows slowly through lymph _____ (very small, irregular channels) within the tissue of the lymph node and is filtered.

70. Lymphatic vessels from all over the body, except the upper right quadrant, drain into the _____, a large lymph vessel that delivers lymph into the base of the left _____ vein.

71. Lymph from lymphatic vessels in the upper right quadrant of the body drains into the right _____, which empties lymph into the base of the right subclavian vein.

Match the term on the left to the correct selection on the right. (Section IV)

72. _____ tonsils

73. _____ spleen

74. _____ lymph node

75. _____ thymus gland

76. _____ palatine

77. _____ macrophages

78. _____ lingual

79. _____ pharyngeal

80. _____ thymosin

A. tonsil located in posterior wall of nasal portion of pharynx above soft palate

B. tonsils that are thickenings in mucous membrane of the throat

C. several hormones collectively produced by thymus gland

D. remove bacteria and other foreign matter from lymph

E. tonsils located at the base of the tongue

F. largest organ of the lymphatic system; filters blood

G. mass of lymph tissue surrounded by a connective tissue capsule

H. masses of lymph tissue located under the epithelial lining of the oral cavity and pharynx

I. pinkish gray lymphatic organ located in the upper thorax

81. Label the parts of the blood circulation in Figure 12-3.

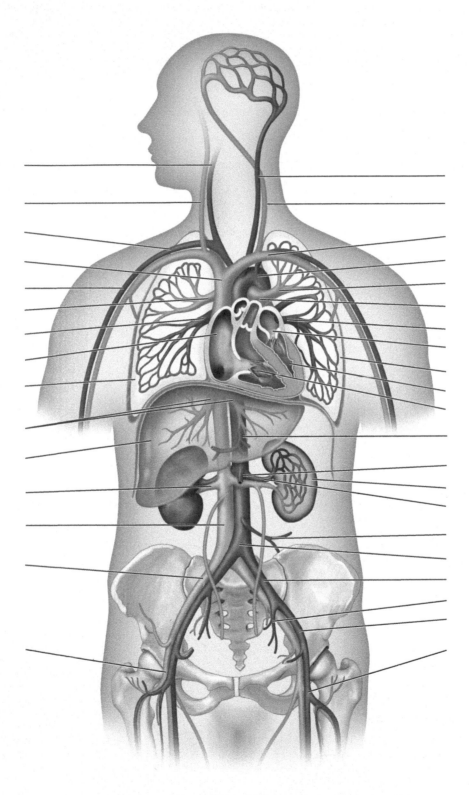

Figure 12-3

82. Label the parts of the aorta and its principal branches in Figure 12-4.

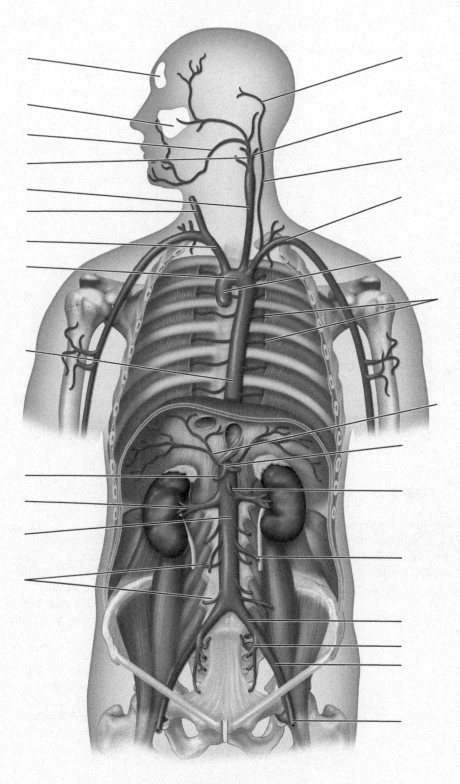

Figure 12-4

Select the correct answer.

1. _____ carries oxygen-rich blood from the

   _____ of the heart to the organs and
   tissues of the body.
   a. Arterioles; atria
   b. An artery; left ventricle
   c. Arteries; atria
   d. Veins; ventricles

2. Small branches of arteries, called _____,
   are important in regulating blood pressure.
   a. venules
   b. capillaries
   c. auricles
   d. arterioles

3. The layers, or tunics, of an artery or vein wall from
   outside to inside are
   a. tunica intima, tunica intima, and tunica adventitia
   b. tunica adventitia, tunica media, and tunica intima
   c. tunica arteriole, tunica intima, and tunica media
   d. tunica adventitia, tunica intima, and tunica media

4. Changes in blood flow are regulated by the

   _____ in response to the metabolic needs
   of the tissue and by the demands of the body.
   a. nervous system
   b. circulatory system
   c. endocrine system
   d. respiratory system

5. Which of the following is *not* a characteristic of
   capillaries?
   a. located close to almost every cell in the body
   b. filter out bacteria in the circulation
   c. permit oxygen and carbon dioxide exchange
      between blood and tissues
   d. wall consists mainly of endothelium

6. Metarterioles are small vessels that directly link
   arterioles with
   a. capillaries
   b. arteries
   c. veins
   d. venules

7. The _____ circulation connects heart

   and lungs and the _____ circulation
   connects the heart with all of the organs and tissues.
   a. pulmonary; systemic
   b. cardiac; pulmonary
   c. systemic; cardiac
   d. systemic; pulmonary

8. The right atrium receives oxygen-poor blood
   returning to the heart from the systemic circulation;
   this blood is pumped into the
   a. left ventricle
   b. left atrium
   c. aorta
   d. right ventricle

9. The right ventricle pumps oxygen-poor blood into

   the _____, which deliver blood to the
   lungs.
   a. pulmonary veins
   b. aorta
   c. venules
   d. pulmonary arteries

10. As blood flows through the pulmonary capillaries,

    _____ diffuses out of the blood as
    oxygen diffuses into it.
    a. carbon dioxide
    b. hemoglobin
    c. lymph
    d. none of the above

11. The _____ return blood, rich in oxygen

    once more, to the _____.
    a. pulmonary veins; left atrium
    b. capillaries; right atrium
    c. pulmonary arteries; left atrium
    d. pulmonary arteries; left ventricle

12. The _____ pumps the blood into the

    _____ and it is pumped into the
    systemic circulation again.
    a. right atrium; right ventricle
    b. right ventricle; left atrium
    c. left atrium; left ventricle
    d. left atrium; right ventricle

Mark each statement true or false; correct the false statements to make them true.

13. _____ The pulmonary veins are the only veins that carry oxygen-rich blood; the pulmonary arteries are the only arteries that transport blood that is poor in oxygen.

14. _____ Blood flow in the pulmonary circulation follows this sequence: right atrium to right ventricle to pulmonary veins; then to pulmonary capillaries to pulmonary arteries to left atrium.

15. _____ The left ventricle pumps the blood into the aorta, which has branches that deliver blood to all the organs and tissues of the body.

16. _____ The superior and inferior venae cavae return blood to the left atrium of the heart.

17. _____ Blood flow to and from the brain is as follows: aorta, common carotid artery, branches of internal carotid artery + basilar artery, circle of Willis, capillaries in brain, venous sinus, internal jugular vein, brachiocephalic vein, superior vena cava.

18. _____ The hepatic portal vein delivers blood from organs of the digestive system to the liver where the blood travels through hepatic sinusoids as liver cells remove/store nutrients and remove toxic substances.

19. _____ Blood pressure is the force exerted by the blood against the inner walls of the blood vessels; it is determined by the flow of blood and the resistance to that flow.

20. _____ Vasoconstriction is a decrease in blood vessel diameter, which decreases resistance to blood flow; vasodilation is an increase in blood vessel diameter, which increases resistance to blood flow.

21. _____ Renin, angiotensin II, and aldosterone are hormones that help regulate blood pressure.

22. _____ The lymph circulation collects excess interstitial fluid and returns it to the blood in the following sequence: lymph capillaries, lymphatic, lymph sinuses in lymph node, lymphatic, thoracic duct (or right lymphatic duct), subclavian vein.

23. _____ Tonsils are masses of lymph tissue located under the epithelial lining of the oral cavity and lungs that filter blood.

24. _____ The spleen, the largest organ of the lymphatic system, filters blood and produces several hormones collectively called thymosin.

PART 3: ACCEPT THE CHALLENGE

1. Would it be more dangerous to suffer a cut to an artery or to a vein? Why?

2. What effect might the lack of gravity in space have on an astronaut's blood circulation?

3. Why are chest compressions so important for people who suffer cardiac arrest?

Find and circle the following words from Chapter 12. Words may be found from top to bottom, bottom to top, right to left, left to right, and diagonally.

```
L O M P F Y Z L R N R A C Z V U Y L E E R E H U Q I S G X Q
J K E X Z M W B X P O O P S Q K M Q X Q U P W C L O M E U E
J W L Y M P H A T I C E U D D V P Z W O O K E D E R W Q S L
N N I H E H L S V Y Y S H U Y D X N B Z O B V E O R I J V O
M H N H U C P E H Y P B U P Z M I Z T K C T L T B H O Z O T
G J Z D V G Q E D U U H D U Y E E O O D C N P Z M P U A T S
D D Q C A R O T I D U R Y D V Q B A X T F E A O B J T V H A
O Y K V P D V M K E B C Y D V C T R T S C U M V W J R B L I
O H C U U A E A D Y M B E Y L I B N H E E K J A D E U X Q D
L R U B L K N X M R R E V I L C I S R C O S O P Y O C H S S
B O W E S Z U Y I F U H Y O D Z Y O B O Q D Y K H M E V D D
L G K D E A L A C E B C M I X U R G L X G J A W B F Y U N M
J S J M D V E U J A U L C B O A F P W E A R T E R Y R L D V
P S P L E E N J L A L J E R B F R S F O L P D K M X A T M A
U E R X I W M R T A Y W R J H T L W S Z N X T V M E L K P S
R Y O K M K R D R J L Z W C B I W Y U H H Q D Z P R L X I O
M L P Y C G Y S A S K F J O S O V P M X T I Y P P F I F T D
F X M E F A R W E A T E Y N L X K V Q I Y H D Q T D P L E I
B A V G G Q N D H C T K O E K J E E D N E R M P J V A P Q L
A H M F S Q I V L R D T C E I G A N U N K D T O T Y C H F A
P Q C G J F Q V M I N V H Y P E R T E N S I O N F A M I C T
Q Q L Q L Y D Q R T J R A R I S V R P B A F Y N P L I V M O
U F Q M Y M A C R O P H A G E D F I J B K B V D L M N D C R
V X X M B A R Z P I N Z F Z V L R C J J V O U Y Y I V T D I
I I M F G M R H M K I D S V C A W L X L Q G W L N X Q J X N
F B W N L I D R U L A I V J L P G E N P D M C E T T Y G S Q
R P G W S E L X M D X J O Y T L J F B P U S R U H V P C V X
W O P N W L G A Z M O C J Z T J T E U Y H K U A G D X W H U
T D K K T G Y Z G V N X Z Y W S K P X E P E O K G X P F V X
A Q C K B V R Z W Z E L O I R E T R A W J W V K V Q U K P Y
```

Artery
Arteriole
Baroreceptor
Blood
Capillary
Carotid
Diastole
Heart
Hypertension
Liver

Lymphatic
Macrophage
Pulse
Renin
Spleen
Tonsils
Vasodilator
Vein
Ventricle
Venule

13 Internal Defense: Immune Responses

LEARNING OBJECTIVES

1. Contrast innate with adaptive immunity.
2. Describe several innate immune responses, including mechanical barriers, phagocytosis, proteins such as cytokines and complement, and the inflammatory response.
3. Identify and give the functions of the principal cells involved in adaptive immune responses.
4. Describe cell-mediated immunity, including the development of memory cells.
5. Describe antibody-mediated immunity, including the effects of antigen-antibody complex on pathogens both directly and through the complement system.
6. Compare primary and secondary immune responses.
7. Contrast active and passive immunity, and give examples of each.
8. Describe three examples of harmful immune responses.

PART 1: LEARN THE TERMS

Match the following terms to the correct definitions by writing the corresponding letter in the space provided. (Section I)

A. adaptive immunity	B. antibodies	C. antigen	D. cell signaling
E. immune response	F. immunological memory	G. immunology	H. innate immunity
I. MHC antigens	J. pathogens		

1. _____ study of internal defense mechanisms

2. _____ organisms that cause disease

3. _____ group of inherited cell-surface proteins

4. _____ system "remembers" foreign or dangerous molecules that it encounters; allows the body to respond faster and more effectively when it encounters the same molecules again

5. _____ recognition of foreign or harmful molecules or abnormal cells and an action aimed at eliminating them

6. _____ highly specific proteins that recognize and bind to specific antigens

7. _____ nonspecific immunity; provides immediate general protection against pathogens

8. _____ any molecule that can be specifically recognized as foreign by cells of the immune system

9. _____ communication among cells

10. _____ specific immunity; provides very specific responses against specific foreign molecules that have entered body

Fill in the blanks with the correct answer for each statement. (Section II)

11. The skin and the _____ that line passageways into the body prevent most pathogens and other harmful substances from entering the body; when pathogens do succeed in penetrating the body, the _____ rapidly responds to destroy them.

12. A large population of harmless _____ inhibit the multiplication of harmful bacteria that happen to land on the skin; sweat and other _____ on the skin's surface contain chemicals that destroy certain types of bacteria.

13. Pathogens that are inhaled may be filtered out by nasal hairs or trapped in the sticky mucous lining of the _____ passageway.

14. Bacteria that enter with food are usually destroyed by acid and enzymes secreted by the _____.

15. A _____ ingests and destroys bacteria, and other foreign matter, by engulfing it; as a bacterium is ingested, it is packaged within a vesicle, and then killed when lysosomes adhere to the vesicle and release _____ into it.

16. _____, the most numerous type of leukocyte, and macrophages are the phagocytes of the immune system.

17. _____ cells (large, granular lymphocytes produced in the bone marrow) recognize and are active against a wide variety of targets, including cells infected with some types of viruses and tumor cells.

18. Natural killer (NK) cells release _____ and enzymes that destroy target cells.

19. _____, located in tissues connected with the outside environment (skin and epithelial linings of the respiratory, digestive, urinary, and vaginal passageways), destroy target cells by both innate and adaptive immune responses.

20. Certain _____ on the cell surface of viruses, certain bacteria, and fungi activate dendritic cells.

Fill in the blanks to correctly complete each sentence, and then unscramble the circled letters to correctly complete the final sentence. (Section II)

21. _ _ ◯ _ _ _ _ ◯ _ are a diverse group of mainly peptides and proteins that cells use to signal one another.

22. Cells secrete cytokines called _ _ _ ◯ _ _ _ ◯ _ _ ◯, when infected by viruses, which interfere with viral replication.

23. Macrophages and certain lymphocytes release _ _ _ ◯ _ _ _ _ _ _ _ ◯ and tumor necrosis factor (TNF) that defend the body against infection.

24. The _ _ ◯ _ _ _ _ ◯ _ system, consisting of more than 20 proteins present in plasma and other body fluids, is important in both innate and adaptive immunity.

25. The inflammatory response brings large numbers of ◯_◯_ _ _ _ _ _ _ _ and proteins to injured or infected areas where pathogens are destroyed, the area is cleaned up, and healing begins.

26. Mast cells release ◯_ _ _◯_ _◯_ and other compounds that dilate blood vessels in the affected area and also make capillaries more permeable.

27. _◯_ _◯◯_ _ _ _ _ _ _ allows increased blood flow to the infected region, bringing great numbers of neutrophils and other phagocytic cells.

28. _◯_◯_ is a common clinical sign of widespread inflammatory response that helps the body fight infection.

29. When pathogens invade tissues, an inflammation develops within a few hours; the clinical characteristics of inflammation are _ _ _ _, _ _ _ _ _ _ _ _ _, _ d _ _ _ _, and _ _ _ _ _.

Match the term on the left to the correct selection on the right. (Section III)

30. _____ T cells	A. responsible for antibody-mediated immunity; they mature into plasma cells
31. _____ monocytes	B. principal combatants in adaptive immune responses
32. _____ antigen-presenting cells	C. gland that makes T cells competent/capable of making immune responses
33. _____ B cells	D. type of immunity carried out by lymphatic system; includes both cell-mediated and antibody-mediated immunity
34. _____ lymphocytes	E. specific surface receptors developed by T cells
35. _____ bone marrow	F. displayed on B cell; binds with specific type of antigen
36. _____ adaptive	G. macrophages and dendritic cells both develop from these white blood cells
37. _____ T-cell receptors	H. display fragments of foreign antigens as well as their own surface proteins to T cells
38. _____ thymus	I. attack body cells infected by invading pathogens, foreign cells, and cells altered by mutation
39. _____ B-cell receptor	J. millions of B cells are produced here daily

Fill in the blanks with the correct answer for each statement. (Section III)

40. When a macrophage ingests a bacterium, some fragments of the foreign _____ are displayed on the surface of the macrophage in association with MHC, a unique molecular identification found on the surface of

each _____.

41. Macrophages, dendritic cells, and _____ function as antigen-presenting cells (APCs), which display fragments of foreign antigens as well as their own surface proteins; the APCs present the displayed antigens to

_____.

42. T cells are responsible for _____ immunity; each T cell is distinguished by a specific

_____ that responds to a specific type of antigen.

43. Cytotoxic T cells, or killer T cells, recognize and destroy cells with foreign antigens on their _____;

killer T cells are also called CD8 cells because they have protein CD8 on the surface of the _____

44. Killer T cells target virus-infected cells, cancer cells, and foreign tissue grafts by releasing a variety of

    _____ and enzymes, which destroy the cells.

45. Helper T cells, also known as _____, secrete cytokines that activate B cells and enhance immune responses.

46. _____ T cells suppress immune responses after pathogens have been destroyed.

47. Some differentiated T cells remain in the _____ as memory T cells for years or decades; if the same

    type of _____ attacks again, the memory cells destroy the invaders so rapidly that they rarely have time to cause symptoms of the disease.

48. B cells are responsible for _____ immunity by producing specific antibodies, also called immunoglobulins, which are highly specific proteins.

49. Immunoglobulins serve as _____ that combine with antigens; only a B cell displaying a matching receptor on its surface can bind a particular antigen.

50. Helper T cells secrete _____ that help activate B cells; activated B cells multiply, and within a few

    days, produce large _____ of identical B cells.

51. Most of the B cell clones mature and become plasma cells that secrete _____, a form of their specific receptor molecule.

52. Unlike killer T cells, plasma cells do not leave the _____; the antibodies secreted by plasma cells are carried by lymph to the blood and are transported to the area of infection.

Match the following terms to the correct definitions by writing the corresponding letter in the space provided. (Sections III, IV)

A. active immunity	B. allergic reaction	C. antigen-antibody	D. graft rejection	E. HIV
F. IgG	G. memory B cells	H. metastasis	I. passive immunity	J. primary
K. secondary	L. tumor			

53. _____ body launches this response the first time it is exposed to a particular antigen

54. _____ borrowed immunity; its effects do not last long; breastfed babies have this

55. _____ 75% of antibodies in the blood belong to this immunoglobulin fraction

56. _____ develops naturally after a particular infection or by immunization

57. _____ activated B cells that continue to produce small amounts of antibody for years

58. _____ spreading of tumor cells to other parts of the body

59. _____ complex that activates several defense mechanisms to fight pathogens

60. _____ body launches this rapid response after second exposure to the same antigen

61. _____ over-function of the immune system

62. _____ virus that causes acquired immunodeficiency syndrome (AIDS)

63. _____ immune response in which T cells destroy the cells of a transplant

64. _____ mass of identical cancer cells

Select the correct answer.

1. Innate and adaptive immunity responses both depend on the body's ability to distinguish
   a. allergies
   b. disease
   c. self from nonself
   d. antibodies

2. Innate immunity provides immediate general protection against
   a. pathogens
   b. antibodies
   c. MHC antigens
   d. allergies

3. Adaptive immunity, or specific immunity, provides very specific responses against specific
   a. interleukins
   b. antibodies
   c. foreign molecules
   d. allergies

4. An adaptive immune response to specific

   _____ is the production of specific

   _____.
   a. antibodies; antigens
   b. diseases; vaccines
   c. antigens; antibodies
   d. allergies; medicines

5. Which of the following would *not* be part of an innate immune response?
   a. phagocytes
   b. T cells
   c. cytokine
   d. complement

6. Which cells are large granular lymphocytes, produced in the bone marrow, that release cytokines and enzymes that destroy cancer cells and cells infected by viruses?
   a. neutrophils
   b. natural killer (NK) cells
   c. plasma cells
   d. dendritic cells

7. _____ are important signaling molecules and have roles in innate and adaptive immune responses.
   a. Cytokines
   b. Antibodies
   c. Vaccines
   d. Leukocytes

8. Which of the following belongs to the diverse group of cytokines?
   a. tumor necrosis factor
   b. interferons
   c. interleukins
   d. all of the above

9. _____ consists of more than 20 proteins present in plasma and other body fluids, and is an important pathogen killer in both innate and adaptive immunity.
   a. Interferon
   b. Complement
   c. Tumor necrosis factor
   d. Cytokines

10. The four clinical characteristics of inflammation during an inflammatory response are
    a. redness, nausea, edema, and heat
    b. edema, heat, bleeding, and nausea
    c. bleeding, nausea, heat, and pain
    d. heat, redness, edema, and pain

11. _____, released by mast cells, causes vasodilation and makes capillaries more permeable.
    a. TNF
    b. Histamine
    c. Interferon
    d. Cytokine

12. Which is *not* a type of lymphocyte involved in immune responses?
    a. T cells
    b. NK cells
    c. neutrophils
    d. B cells

13. All of the following is true concerning T cells *except*
    a. responsible for antibody-mediated immunity
    b. originate from stem cells in the bone marrow
    c. mature in the thymus gland
    d. attack invading pathogens and foreign cells

14. All of the following is true concerning B cells *except*
    a. responsible for antibody-mediated immunity
    b. produced in the thymus gland
    c. mature into plasma cells that produce specific antibodies
    d. leave the bone marrow to mature in the fetal liver

Mark each statement true or false; correct the false statements to make them true.

15. _____ B cells and T cells are found in the spleen, lymph nodes, tonsils, and other lymphatic tissues strategically positioned throughout the body.

16. _____ Macrophages, dendritic cells, and T cells function as APCs, which display fragments of foreign antigens as well as their own surface proteins.

17. _____ Killer T cells, also called CD8 cells, kill their target cells by releasing a variety of cytokines and enzymes that destroy cells.

18. _____ Regulatory T cells, also called CD4 cells, secrete cytokines that activate B cells and enhance immune responses; helper T cells suppress immune responses after pathogens have been destroyed.

19. _____ Cell-mediated immunity follows the sequence: virus infects body, APCs display foreign antigen from virus, specific T cells are activated, activated T cells multiply forming clones of activated T cells, killer T cells migrate to infected area, release enzymes that destroy the pathogens.

20. _____ Antibody-mediated immunity occurs this way: pathogen infects body, APCs present foreign antigen to helper T cells, activated helper T cells activate B cells with receptors that match antigen, activated B cells multiply, clones of activated B cells, most develop into plasma cells, plasma cells secrete antibodies, antibodies are transported to infected area, antibodies destroy pathogens.

21. _____ The principal job of an antibody is to identify a pathogen as foreign by combining with the matching antigen on the surface of the pathogen.

22. _____ The antigen-antibody complex activates several defense mechanisms including phagocytes and antibodies of the IgG and IgM groups, which activate the complement system.

23. _____ In active immunity, an individual is given antibodies actively produced by other humans or by animals. Passive immunity is borrowed immunity, so its effects do not last long.

24. _____ Cancer cells have abnormal surface lipids that the immune system targets for destruction by NK cells, macrophages, and B cells; often antigens stimulate weak, ineffective immune responses allowing cancer cells to evade the immune system and multiply unchecked.

25. _____ Transplanted organs have foreign antigens that stimulate graft rejection, an immune response in which T cells destroy the cells of the transplant.

PART 3: ACCEPT THE CHALLENGE

1. How would a body respond to a pathogen if it did not have the ability to distinguish self from nonself?

2. How do major burns reduce the functional ability of the immune system?

3. Why does a person bitten by a venomous snake need to receive a specific antivenom, immunoglobulin, to recover?

Answer the questions to complete the crossword puzzle.

Body Plays Defense

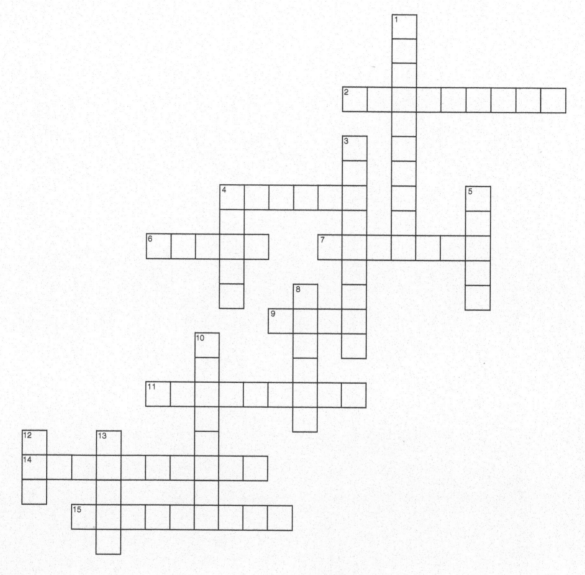

Across

2. surrounds and consumes pathogens
4. gland that makes T cells competent
6. sign of widespread inflammatory response that helps body fight infection
7. borrowed immunity
9. a clinical characteristic of inflammation; ouch!
11. organisms that cause disease
14. study of the body's internal defense mechanisms
15. macrophages and dendritic cells develop from these cells

Down

1. spread of tumor cells to other parts of body
3. causes vasodilation and makes capillaries more permeable
4. responsible for cell-mediated immunity
5. responsible for antibody-mediated immunity
8. disease that sometimes evades immune system and multiplies unchecked
10. highly specific protein that recognizes and binds to specific antigens
12. virus that causes AIDS
13. mass of identical cancer cells

14 The Respiratory System

CHAPTER GUIDE

I. The respiratory system consists of the airway and lungs
    A. The nasal cavities are lined with a mucous membrane
    B. The pharynx is divided into three regions
    C. The larynx contains the vocal cords
    D. The trachea is supported by rings of cartilage
    E. The primary bronchi enter the lungs

F. The lungs provide a large surface area for gas exchange
II. Ventilation moves air into and out of the lungs
III. Gas exchange occurs by diffusion
IV. Gases are transported by the circulatory system
V. Respiration is regulated by the brain
VI. The respiratory system defends itself against polluted air

LEARNING OBJECTIVES

1. Trace a breath of air through the respiratory system from nostrils to alveoli.
2. Describe the structure and function of each of the respiratory organs.
3. Contrast inspiration and expiration.
4. Compare the process of gas exchange in the lungs with gas exchange in the tissues.

5. Compare the transport of oxygen and carbon dioxide in the blood.
6. Describe how the body regulates respiration.
7. Describe defense mechanisms that protect the lungs from air pollutants and describe some effects of breathing dirty air.

PART 1: LEARN THE TERMS

Match the following terms to the correct definitions by writing the corresponding letter in the space provided. (Section I)

A. airway   B. alveoli   C. larynx   D. nasal conchae   E. nasal septum
F. nostrils   G. paranasal sinuses   H. pharynx   I. respiration   J. respiratory system
K. trachea

1. _____ exchange of gases between the body and its environment

2. _____ openings into the nose; nares

3. _____ voice box

4. _____ microscopic air sacs

5. _____ consists of the lungs and the airway

6. _____ series of tubes through which air flows to and from air sacs of the lungs

7. _____ partition separating the two nasal cavities

8. _____ small cavities in the bones of the skull connected with the nasal cavities

9. _____ windpipe

10. _____ they increase surface area over which air passes as it moves through the nose

11. _____ throat

Fill in the blanks with the correct answer for each statement. (Section I)

12. Air enters the _____, the superior part of the pharynx, and then moves down into the oropharynx

    behind the _____.

13. Air passes through the laryngopharynx and enters the opening into the _____, called the glottis.

14. The wall of the larynx is supported by _____ protruding from the midline of the neck, sometimes
    referred to as the Adam's apple.

15. The _____, muscular folds of tissue that project into the larynx from its lateral walls, vibrate as air

    from the _____ rushes past them during expiration (breathing out).

16. A flap of tissue, the _____, automatically closes off the larynx during swallowing so that food and
    water do not enter the lower airway; foreign matter that does come into contact with the sensitive larynx

    stimulates a _____ to expel the material from the respiratory system.

17. The _____, or windpipe, is located anterior to the esophagus and extends from the larynx to the middle

    of the chest; it is supported by C-shaped rings of _____ in its wall.

18. The _____ keeps foreign matter out of the lungs by the action of ciliated cells lining the larynx,
    trachea, and bronchi, which continuously beat a stream of mucus upward to the pharynx where it is swallowed.

19. The _____ divides into right and left primary (main) bronchi; one bronchus enters each lung, and

    inside the lung, each _____ branches repeatedly, and is referred to as the bronchial tree.

20. Branches give rise to increasingly smaller bronchi and then to very small _____; each

    _____ has more than 1 million bronchioles.

Match the term on the left to the correct selection on the right. (Section I)

21. _____ hilus   A. middle part of thoracic cavity; contains the heart, esophagus, thymus gland

22. _____ parietal pleura   B. depression where blood vessels and nerves enter and leave the lung

23. _____ pleural membrane   C. large paired organs that occupy the thoracic cavity

24. _____ pulmonary surfactant   D. strong, dome-shaped muscle; floor of thoracic cavity

25. _____ visceral pleura   E. space between the visceral and parietal pleura

26. _____ alveoli   F. thin film that coats alveoli; prevents lungs from collapsing

27. _____ lungs   G. portion of the pleural membrane that lines thoracic cavity

28. _____ mediastinum   H. cluster of microscopic air sacs

29. _____ diaphragm   I. forms a sac enclosing the lungs and continues as a lining of the thoracic
                                         cavity

30. _____ pleural cavity   J. part of the pleural membrane that covers the lungs

Fill in the blanks with the correct answer for each statement. (Section II)

31. We normally breathe by the process of _____, the movement of air into and out of the lungs.

32. _____, or inhalation, is the process of taking air into the lungs (breathing in); _____, or
    exhalation, is the process of breathing out.

33. During inspiration, the _____ contracts, flattens, and moves downward; external intercostal muscles also contract pulling each _____ up and out.

34. As these actions increase the size of the chest cavity, the film of fluid on the _____ holds the lung surfaces against the chest wall and the lungs expand along with the chest wall; the space within each lung _____.

35. The pressure of the air in the lungs falls below the air pressure outside the _____ creating a partial vacuum; this causes outside air to rush in through the respiratory _____ and fill the lungs until the two pressures are again equal.

36. _____ occurs as the diaphragm and external intercostal muscles relax, permitting the elastic lung tissues to recoil; the size of the _____ decreases, increasing the pressure inside the lungs.

37. As pressure _____, elastic fibers push against the air, forcing it to rush out of the lungs; millions of _____ deflate and the lungs are ready for another inspiration.

38. The pressure between the visceral and parietal pleura is lower than _____; this difference prevents the air sacs from completely deflating at the end of each _____.

Unscramble each term and match it to its correct description. (Section III)

39. olliave

40. fnoudifsi

41. nyolpmuar

42. tayrlcciruo

43. bncaro xoeidid

44. gusln

A. diffuses in from the blood to the alveoli as oxygen diffuses out

B. vital system linking alveoli and the body cells for oxygen transport

C. oxygen diffuses from here into the blood

D. carbon dioxide diffuses from cells into the blood and is transported here

E. net movement of molecules from a region of higher concentration to a region of lower concentration

F. oxygen is loaded into the blood in the _____ capillaries

Match the following terms to the correct definitions by writing the corresponding letter in the space provided. (Section IV)

A. bicarbonate   B. carbonic acid   C. chemical buffer   D. circulatory
E. hemoglobin   F. oxygen   G. oxyhemoglobin   H. red blood cells

45. _____ oxyhemoglobin easily dissociates to hemoglobin and this gas

46. _____ most carbon dioxide in the blood is transported as these ions

47. _____ most hydrogen ions released from carbonic acid combine with this compound

48. _____ oxygen diffuses into the blood and enters these cells

49. _____ substance that lessens the change in hydrogen ion concentration

50. _____ in plasma, carbon dioxide slowly combines with water to form this

51. _____ red blood cells and hemoglobin form weak chemical bonds to produce this

52. _____ oxygen and carbon dioxide are transported in the blood by this system

Chapter 14 The Respiratory System

Fill in the blanks with the correct answer for each statement. (Sections V, VI)

53. _____is a rhythmic, involuntary process regulated by respiratory centers in the brainstem, specifically

    groups of neurons in the dorsal region of the _____.

54 The neurons send a burst of impulses to the _____ by way of phrenic nerves and to the external

    intercostal muscles by way of _____, causing them to contract.

55. Respiratory centers in the pons help control the transition from inspiration to expiration, which can stimulate or

    inhibit the _____ in the medulla.

56. A group of neurons in the _____ region of the medulla becomes active only when we need to breathe
    forcefully.

57. Specialized _____ in the medulla are sensitive to changes in carbon dioxide concentration, the most
    important chemical stimulus for regulating the rate of respiration.

58. When stimulated, chemoreceptors signal _____, leading to increases in both breathing rate and depth
    of breathing; as carbon dioxide is removed by the lungs, hydrogen ion concentration in the extracellular fluid

    decreases and the body returns to _____.

59. Underwater swimmers and some Asian pearl divers purposefully _____ before going under water by

    taking a series of deep inhalations and exhalations; they "blow off" _____ reducing the content in
    alveolar air and blood, which extends the time before needing to breathe.

60. When we breathe dirty air, the _____ narrow; this bronchial constriction increases the chances that

    inhaled particles land on sticky mucous linings of the respiratory _____.

61. Chain smokers, and those who breathe heavily polluted air, may live in a chronic state of _____.

62. Foreign particles that slip through respiratory defenses and reach the alveoli may be engulfed by _____

    or may remain there indefinitely; macrophages themselves may accumulate in _____ of the lungs.

63. Chronic smokers and people who regularly breathe dirty air may have large, blackened areas of lung tissue where

    _____ have been deposited; chronic bronchitis and _____ are chronic pulmonary diseases
    that can result from continued exposure.

64. _____ is the main cause of lung cancer due to carcinogenic compounds in tobacco smoke, which
    transform normal cells into cancer cells.

65. Label the parts of the respiratory system in Figure 14-1.

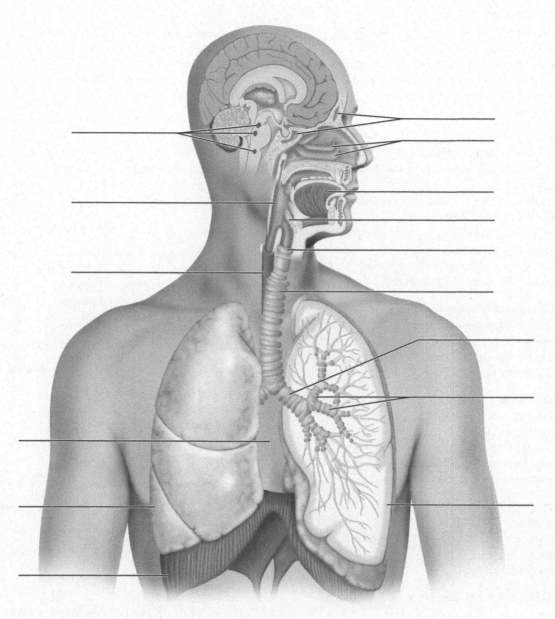

Figure 14-1

Select the correct answer.

1. Which of the following is *not* a function of the respiratory system?
   a. gas exchange between the lungs and the blood
   b. gas exchange between the blood and the cells
   c. circulation of blood and lymph
   d. breathing

2. Which is the correct sequence for a breath of air moving from nostrils to alveoli?
   a. pharynx, trachea, larynx, primary bronchioles, and alveoli
   b. nasal cavities, larynx, pharynx, primary bronchus, pulmonary artery, and alveoli
   c. nasal cavities, capillaries, larynx, pharynx, bronchioles, and alveoli
   d. nasal cavities, pharynx, larynx, trachea, primary bronchus, bronchioles, and alveoli

3. Which functions occur in the nasal cavity?
   a. air is filtered and moistened
   b. receptors detect odors
   c. mucus produced here traps foreign materials
   d. all of the above

4. The parts of the pharynx in order, beginning at the nasal cavities, are
   a. nasopharynx, oropharynx, laryngopharynx
   b. laryngopharynx, nasopharynx, oropharynx
   c. laryngopharynx, larynx, nasopharynx
   d. oropharynx, nasopharynx, larynx

5. The opening into the larynx is the
   a. epiglottis
   b. glottis
   c. trachea
   d. vocal cords

6. The trachea is located anterior to the

   _____ and extends from the

   _____ to the middle of the chest.
   a. esophagus; nasal cavities
   b. esophagus; larynx
   c. larynx; nasal cavities
   d. nasal cavities; esophagus

7. The network of branching air passageways within the lungs is referred to as the
   a. bronchial tree
   b. cilia-propelled mucus elevator
   c. respiratory system
   d. alveoli

8. Which of the following enters the lung at the hilus?
   a. blood vessels
   b. primary bronchus
   c. nerves
   d. all of the above

9. The _____ covers the lung and the

   _____ line(s) the thoracic cavity.
   a. visceral pleura; ciliated epithelial cells
   b. parietal pleura; visceral pleura
   c. visceral pleura; parietal pleura
   d. visceral pleura; diaphragm

10. The wall of an alveolus consists of a single layer of

    _____ and elastic fibers, and is

    surrounded by a network of _____.
    a. mucus; epithelial cells
    b. epithelial cells; nerves
    c. epithelial cells; capillaries
    d. capillaries; nerves

11. A premature baby with underdeveloped lungs may

    lack _____ to help prevent the lungs
    from collapsing.
    a. alveoli
    b. pulmonary surfactant
    c. capillaries
    d. mucus

12. Which of the following is the floor of the thoracic cavity?
    a. visceral pleura
    b. diaphragm
    c. abdomen
    d. pleural membrane

Mark each statement true or false; correct the false statements to make them true.

13. _____ Pulmonary ventilation is normally accomplished by inspiration and expiration.

14. _____ The thoracic cavity is open at both ends, so that air can enter and pass through the trachea.

15. _____ The sequence for inspiration is: diaphragm and external intercostal muscles contract, volume of chest cavity increases, lungs expand, volume of lungs increases, air pressure in lungs decreases, air moves into lungs.

16. _____ The sequence for expiration is: diaphragm and intercostal muscles relax, volume of thoracic cavity increases, lungs recoil, lung volume increases, pressure in alveoli increases, air rushes out of lungs.

17. _____ Because the alveoli contain a greater concentration of oxygen than the blood entering the pulmonary capillaries, oxygen molecules diffuse from the alveoli into the blood.

18. _____ When carbon dioxide is more concentrated in the cells than in the blood, it diffuses from the cells into the blood and is transported to the lungs.

19. _____ Carbon dioxide is transported in the blood by being dissolved in air, attached to hemoglobin, and as carbonic acid.

20. _____ Hemoglobin is a very effective chemical buffer that lessens the change in hydrogen ion concentration in the blood.

21. _____ Carbon dioxide concentration is the most important chemical stimulus for regulating the rate of respiration and is regulated by specialized chemoreceptors in the medulla.

22. _____ Respiratory centers in the pons help control the transition from inspiration to expiration by stimulating or inhibiting the respiratory centers in the medulla.

23. _____ Cigarette smoking decreases bronchial restriction and can lead to chronic bronchitis and emphysema.

PART 3: ACCEPT THE CHALLENGE

1. Why does the body produce more mucus during infections and allergic reactions?

2. How do you think sudden lung collapse is treated?

3. How would carbon monoxide inhalation affect the body? Note that carbon monoxide (CO) binds to the same binding sites on hemoglobin as oxygen (O_2). However, hemoglobin has a much greater affinity for CO than for oxygen. When CO binds to hemoglobin, the hemoglobin cannot bind with O_2.

Find and circle the following words from Chapter 12. Words may be found from top to bottom, bottom to top, right to left, left to right, and diagonally.

```
F J V X N I S U K M B Z N Z M G D M W D D P D R O K R H E O
N O B Q T L O U T Y W N K K U O I M X Q U J O X O D C H T M
Y C T P Q H Q G L B D W W E N U A J Q E Z C B R Y N F W D L
Y L G N J J G A Z I N R H Q I W P G O C A Z T H Z X K S Y X
Y U B L U O T J Z C H R A D T H H T N X P T O U V N P E M M
P F E K O F G R A S D F L O S F R Q G F V N Y I M P D A J B
Q Y X F E N W E L Z L Q I C A K A N I Y B N Q H U L W U W L
J B P N V E H D V K I K I T I K G T M U W Y H G W I V M S P
A O I J W C B U Z P R E S M D N M Q C X Y W J S K D Q I K W
H T R T A V N I V B T T U D E P T U H Z M U P R T P P D J Z
G Z A R S J T X S O Q C O B M A J E V F H L A B S Z Q O O H
J F T W G M I P X V U Q B R O N C H I O L E S I Q O B E G P
F H I A N J L C F S T P F W J E O Z U X J A V X R S U H D K
V E O O U E O V V L V H P D C F K A C Q P P Q L M Z N I Y G
Y C N T L O E I H D L L U P L E U R A L P I P C E Y S J A Z
R T B P K S V H H W E I L O H S T A R G T H O R A C I C A D
A T O X J D L W P C L C N F L Q G F T T W P L F N L P O Z G
N V T B V I A B B A N U P A F O P R I Q E Y C U F A H N D Y
O A I M S F Y N Y T G O Z Q J C R F L U R X L I I R E Y M C
M C J J L F Y M K Z X W R T V L R R A R S H N C W Y A H Q T
L S Y B Y U Z Q B B Z M N B Z B Z A G Y V T V Y G N M M Z E
U U D D U S K T O F U R D V H G Y I E T L I W M R X K U H E
P P P Q C E Q R E S P I R A T I O N X Y T C U G V A K N R C
Q M L Z L U U Y E Q L O M U U B K N F C M F Y O A E H J K R
B O J P A I A U E Z A U K O G E L K Q Y R V M X T A Z P X L
J Q O Y B E Y K E U Q F U L P K T W V F O V X J H W C J V B
V E O X Y G E N E H T A E R B T J E V P E H W Y X B U K T F
G R C L F A K P H G T T D V O K Q Z O L P T S L T S O O C H
V K Y X Y E X I V H R Q A U N Q E E P V P G Q K T J C I Z G
R U T Q S R W R Z T Y S J A N X Q R B I O S Q E C K O G U P
```

Alveoli	Lungs
Breathe	Mediastinum
Bronchi	Mucus
Bronchioles	Oxygen
Cartilage	Pharynx
Diaphragm	Pleural
Diffuse	Pulmonary
Expiration	Respiration
Hilus	Trachea
Larynx	Thoracic

15 The Digestive System

CHAPTER GUIDE

I. The digestive system processes food
   A. The wall of the digestive tract has four layers
   B. Folds of the peritoneum support the digestive organs
II. Structures of the digestive system have specific functions
   A. The mouth ingests food
      1. The teeth break down food
      2. The salivary glands produce saliva
   B. The pharynx is important in swallowing
   C. The esophagus conducts food to the stomach
   D. The stomach digests proteins
   E. Most digestion takes place in the small intestine

F. The pancreas secretes enzymes
G. The liver secretes bile
III. Food is digested as it moves through the digestive tract
   A. Glucose is the main product of carbohydrate digestion
   B. Bile emulsifies fat
   C. Proteins are digested to free amino acids
IV. Absorption takes place through the intestinal villi
V. The large intestine eliminates wastes
VI. A balanced diet is necessary to maintain health
VII. Energy metabolism is balanced when energy input is equal to energy output

LEARNING OBJECTIVES

1. Describe in general terms the following steps in processing food: ingestion, digestion, absorption, and elimination.
2. List in sequence each structure through which a bite of food passes on its way through the digestive tract; label a diagram of the digestive system.
3. Describe the wall of the digestive tract; distinguish between the visceral and parietal peritoneum, and describe their major folds.
4. Describe the structures of the mouth, including the teeth, and give their functions.
5. Connect the structure and function of the esophagus.
6. Connect the structure of the stomach with its functions.
7. Identify the three main regions of the small intestine, and connect its structure with its functions.

8. Describe the functions of the pancreas and liver.
9. Summarize carbohydrate, lipid, and protein digestion.
10. Connect the structure of intestinal villi with their function in absorption of nutrients.
11. Describe the structure and functions of the large intestine.
12. Describe the components of a balanced diet and summarize the functions of each.
13. Contrast basal metabolic rate with total metabolic rate, and write the basic equation for maintaining body weight.
14. Describe the effects of malnutrition, including both undernutrition and overnutrition.

PART 1: LEARN THE TERMS

Match the following terms to the correct definitions by writing the corresponding letter in the space provided. (Section I)

A. absorption	B. alimentary canal	C. chemical	D. digestion
E. digestive system	F. elimination	G. enzyme	H. gastrointestinal (GI) tract
I. ingestion	J. mechanical	K. nutrients	L. nutrition

1. _____ substances in food that the body uses

2. _____ taking food into mouth, chewing it, and swallowing it

3. _____ removal of undigested and unabsorbed food from the body

4. _____ transport of digested food through the stomach wall or intestine and into the circulatory system

5. _____ process of taking in and using food

6. _____ digestion by breaking down large molecules, such as carbohydrates, proteins, and fats, into smaller molecules that can be absorbed from the digestive tract and used by cells

7. _____ system that digests food, breaking it down into small molecules and ions for absorption and delivery to cells

8. _____ chemical catalyst, typically a specific protein

9. _____ breakdown of food into smaller molecules

10. _____ digestion process of breaking down pieces of food by chewing, and by churning and mixing movements in the stomach

11. _____ 8 m tube extending from mouth to anus; digestive tract

12. _____ digestive tract below the diaphragm

Unscramble the parts of the digestive tract and put them in order, beginning with the mouth. (Section I)

grela itstinnee   xyarnhp   snau   pseogshau   umtho   mlsal esentinti   camshto

13. _____

14. _____

15. _____

16. _____

17. _____

18. _____

19. _____

Fill in the blanks with the correct answer for each statement. (Section I)

20. The three types of accessory digestive glands are the salivary glands, _____, and pancreas; they are not part of the digestive tract but secrete _____ into it.

21. The wall of the digestive tract consists of four main layers from the _____ to the anus.

22. The _____, the lining of the digestive tract, consists of epithelial tissue resting on a layer of loose _____ tissue.

23. The _____ is specialized in different areas for protection of underlying tissues, secretion of mucus or digestive juices, or absorption of nutrients; the mucosa is repeatedly folded in the stomach and _____, significantly increasing surface area for digestion and absorption.

24. The _____, rich in blood vessels and nerves, is a layer of connective tissue beneath the mucosa.

25. A muscle layer (muscularis), surrounding the submucosa, consists of two sublayers of _____; the muscle contracts in a wavelike motion, called _____, that pushes food along through the digestive tract.

26. The outer layer of the digestive tract wall consists of _____, called the _____ above the diaphragm level and called the visceral peritoneum below the level of the diaphragm.

27. Various folds connect the visceral peritoneum to the _____, a sheet of connective tissue lining the walls of the abdominal and pelvic cavities; the peritoneal _____ is a potential space between the visceral and the parietal peritoneum.

28. The _____, a large fan-shaped double-fold of peritoneal tissue, extends from the parietal peritoneum and attaches to the _____.

29. The mesentery anchors the intestine to the posterior _____.

30. The _____ (fatty apron) is a large double-fold of peritoneum attached to the stomach and intestine that hangs down over the intestine; it contains large fat deposits and _____ that help protect the peritoneum from infection.

31. The lesser omentum suspends the stomach and _____ from the liver; another fold of peritoneum, the _____, attaches the colon to the posterior abdominal wall.

Match the term on the left to the correct selection on the right. (Section II)

32. _____ teeth	A. tooth area above the gum
33. _____ mouth	B. pushes food about to aid chewing and swallowing; oral cavity
34. _____ enamel	C. posterior teeth modified for grinding and crushing
35. _____ root	D. break down food mechanically; adults have 32
36. _____ pulp	E. adult teeth; 32 in number
37. _____ crown	F. ingests food and begins the process of digestion
38 _____ tongue	G. calcified connective tissue; imparts shape and rigidity to teeth
39. _____ root canal	H. tooth area beneath the gum line
40. _____ dentin	I. tough covering on a tooth crown
41. _____ deciduous	J. passes through the root of the tooth
42. _____ molars	K. 20 in number; full set present by about 2 years of age
43. _____ permanent	L. specialized for biting and cutting
44. _____ canine	M. extremely sensitive connective tissue containing blood vessels and nerves
45. _____ incisors	N. assist incisors in biting

46. Label the parts of the tooth in Figure 15-1.

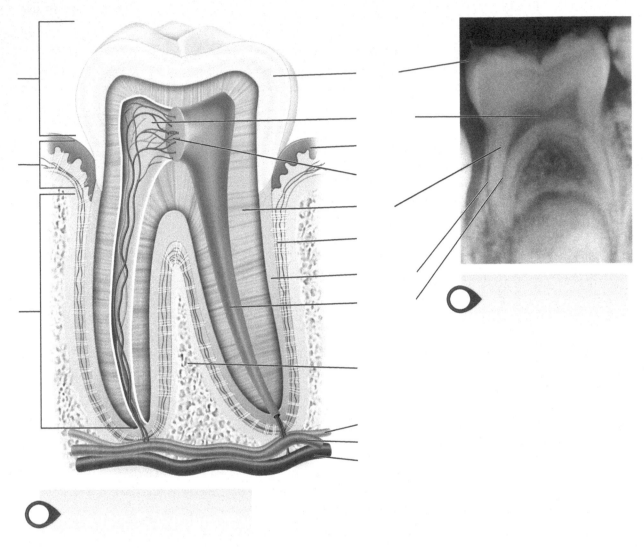

Figure 15-1

Fill in the blanks with the correct answer for each statement. (Section II)

47. The salivary glands produce saliva, which consists of the following: a thin, watery secretion containing

_____, a digestive enzyme that begins the chemical digestion of starches (large carbohydrates), and a

mucus secretion that _____ the mouth.

48. Saliva lubricates the tissues of the mouth and _____, making it easier to talk and chew; saliva helps the

tongue convert a mouthful of food to a semisolid mass called a _____ that can be easily swallowed.

49. The _____, located in the tissue inferior and anterior to the ears, are the largest salivary glands.

50. The smaller submandibular glands lie below the _____; the _____ are located under the
tongue.

51. During swallowing, the bolus is forced into the _____ by the tongue; the opening to the larynx is closed by the epiglottis, a small flap of tissue that prevents food from entering the _____ passageways.

52. The oropharynx and nasopharynx are partitioned by the muscular _____, which hangs down between them.

53. The soft palate is a posterior extension of the bony _____, the roof of the mouth; the _____ a small mass of tissue, hangs from the lower border of the soft palate.

54. The opening to the larynx is closed during swallowing by the _____, a small flap of tissue that prevents food from entering the respiratory passageways.

55. Reflex contractions of muscles in the pharynx and esophageal walls, called _____, propel the bolus through the pharynx and then the esophagus, which passes through the diaphragm and empties into the

_____

56. When a peristaltic wave passes down the esophagus, the _____ muscle relaxes and permits the bolus to enter the stomach.

Match the following terms to the correct definitions by writing the corresponding letter in the space provided. (Section II)

A. chyme	**B. gastric glands**	**C. hydrochloric acid**	**D. intrinsic factor**	**E. parietal cells**
F. pepsin	**G. pepsinogen**	**H. pyloric sphincter**	**I. rugae**	**J. stomach**

57. _____ extend deep into the stomach wall; contain parietal cells

58. _____ needed for adequate absorption of vitamin B_{12}

59. _____ enzyme that begins digestion of proteins

60. _____ large muscular organ that mashes and churns food

61. _____ strong ring of muscle at the exit of the stomach

62. _____ folds in lining of empty stomach

63. _____ secreted by chief cells

64. _____ secrete hydrochloric acid and intrinsic factor

65. _____ kills bacteria and breaks down connective tissues in meat

66. _____ soupy mixture of converted food

Fill in the blanks with the correct answer for each statement. (Section II)

67. Most digestion takes place in the _____, a long coiled tube more than 5 to 6 m long by 4 cm in diameter; the first 22 cm of the small intestine make up the _____, which is curved like the letter C.

68. The small intestine is called the _____ as it turns downward, extending for about 2 m; the third part of the small intestine, the _____ is about 3.5 m long.

69. _____ are tiny fingerlike projections that line the small intestine; millions of these structures increase the _____ of the small intestine increasing the digestion and absorption of nutrients.

70. The intestinal lining is further expanded by _____, tiny projections of the plasma membrane of each of the epithelial cells of the villi.

71. _____ extend downward into the mucosa between adjacent villi; these glands secrete large amounts of fluid to help keep the _____ in a fluid state so that nutrients can be easily absorbed.

72. Goblet cells in the mucosa secrete _____ mucus, which helps protect the intestinal wall from the acidic chyme and from the action of digestive _____.

73. Most digestion takes place in the _____; the liver and pancreas release digestive juices into the duodenum where enzymes produced in the epithelial cell lining complete the job of breaking down food molecules for _____.

74. The _____ is a large long gland that lies in the abdomen posterior to the stomach; the pancreatic duct from the pancreas joins the _____ duct leaving the liver to form a single duct that enters into the duodenum.

75. The pancreas is both an endocrine and an _____ gland; its endocrine cells secrete the hormones insulin and glucagon, which regulate _____; the exocrine portion secretes pancreatic juice, which contains a number of digestive enzymes.

Match the term on the left to the correct selection on the right. (Section II)

76. _____ common bile duct   A. delivers nutrients absorbed from the intestine

77. _____ liver   B. bile is stored and concentrated here

78. _____ bilirubin   C. hormone stimulates the gallbladder to contract and release bile

79. _____ hepatic artery   D. secretion important in the mechanical digestion of fats

80. _____ bile   E. largest organ inside the body; secretes bile

81. _____ gall bladder   F. cystic duct from the gallbladder and hepatic duct from the liver form this

82. _____ cholecystokinin   G. brings oxygen-rich blood to the liver

83. _____ hepatic portal vein   H. released from hemoglobin and secreted into bile

Unscramble each term and match it to its correct description. (Section III)

84. lastmoe   A. large carbohydrates (starch and glycogen) consist of long chains of this molecule

85. tcaepcrani ysamlae   B. enzyme that breaks down starch

86. luselolec   C. breaks maltose down to glucose

87. sclguoe   D. starch is broken down into smaller carbohydrates and this sugar

88. slemata   E. sucrose and lactose are broken down to simple sugars here

89. vilysaar laasyme   F. enzyme in pancreatic juice that splits remaining starch molecules to maltose

90. umuodden   G. indigestible starch in the cell walls of plants

Fill in the blanks with the correct answer for each statement. (Section III, IV)

91. Digestion of fat takes place mainly in the duodenum where bile _____ fat by a detergent action breaking large fat droplets down into smaller droplets.

92. _____ breaks down triglycerides, or fat molecules, to free fatty acids and glycerol.

93. During protein digestion _____ are broken and free amino acids are released.

94. Protein digestion begins in the _____ where pepsin breaks down most proteins to smaller _____.

95. In the duodenum, _____ and other enzymes in the pancreatic juice break down proteins and polypeptides to smaller _____.

96. Peptides are digested by enzymes called _____ secreted by intestinal epithelial cells; peptidases split peptides into _____, the end products of protein digestion.

97. Digestion is regulated by _____ and hormones through neural messages sent to the GI tract by way of sympathetic and parasympathetic nerves.

98. The four major GI hormones gastrin, secretin, cholecystokinin (CCK), and glucose-dependent insulinotropic peptide (GIP) are important in regulating _____.

99. Each villus contains a network of _____ that branch from an arteriole and empty into a venule; each villus also has a central _____ called a lacteal.

100. After food is digested, _____ must pass through a single layer of epithelial cells lining the villus and through a single layer of cells forming the wall of a capillary to reach the blood, or through a _____ to reach the lymph.

Match the following terms to the correct definitions by writing the corresponding letter in the space provided. (Section V)

A. anus	B. ascending colon	C. cecum	D. colon	E. defecate
F. descending colon	G. ileocecal valve	H. microbiome	I. rectum	J. transverse colon
K. vermiform appendix				

101. _____ extends across the abdomen below the liver and stomach

102. _____ part of the large intestine from cecum to rectum

103. _____ last 12 cm of the digestive tract; includes the anal canal

104. _____ expel feces

105. _____ worm-shaped blind tube, hangs down from the end of the cecum

106. _____ all of the microorganisms that live on or in the body

107. _____ pouch where the small and large intestine join

108. _____ turns downward and empties into the S-shaped sigmoid colon

109. _____ extends from the cecum straight up to the lower border of liver

110. _____ sphincter muscle controlling chyme flow into the large intestine

111. _____ opening for elimination of feces; end of the digestive tract

Fill in the blanks to correctly complete each sentence, and then unscramble the circled letters to correctly complete the final sentence. (Section VI)

112. _ O _ _ _ is an essential component of the body because all of the body's chemical reactions take place in a watery medium and it is needed to transport materials.

113. _ O _ _ _ _ _ _ are inorganic nutrients ingested in the form of salts dissolved in food and water; many minerals are necessary components of body tissues and fluids.

114. Vitamins are organic compounds required for certain chemical reactions; many vitamins act as

   _ O _ O _ _ _ _ O, compounds that work with enzymes to regulate chemical reactions.

115. _ O _ _ _ _ _ O _ _ O _ _ are ingested mainly as starch or cellulose (both polysaccharides), which are complex carbohydrates; polysaccharides are digested to glucose or other simple sugars that can be absorbed into the blood.

116. _ O _ _ _ _, including fats and cholesterol, provide energy and are needed to make cell membranes, steroid hormones, and bile salts.

117. _ _ _ O _ _ O _ are digested into their component amino acids and then reassembled to make the types of proteins the body needs; nine amino acids are considered essential because they must be provided in the diet.

118. Phytochemicals are biologically active plant compounds that function as _ _ _ _ _ x _ _ _ _ _ _, substances that destroy DNA-damaging oxidants.

Fill in the blanks with the correct answer for each statement. (Section VII)

119. _____ is the amount of energy released by the body in a given time as a result of breaking down fuel

   molecules; much of the energy expended by the body is ultimately converted to _____.

120. The _____ is the rate at which the body releases heat at rest; it is the body's basic cost of living, or

   maintaining body _____, such as heart contraction, breathing, and kidney function.

121. An individual's total _____ is the sum of the BMR and the energy used to carry on all daily activities.

122. The _____ regulates energy metabolism and food intake; the GI tract, fat cells, and the pancreas release compounds signaling the hypothalamus about nutritional status.

123. _____ is a poor nutritional status, which can result from a dietary intake that is more or less than what is required.

124. Millions of people suffer from _____ in which their calorie, or energy, intake is too low or their diet is deficient in essential nutrients.

125. _____, especially in more affluent regions of the world is a serious health problem; consuming too

   many calories and not expending an equal amount of energy can result in _____ with excess fat deposited all over the body.

126. Label the parts of the digestive system in Figure 15-2

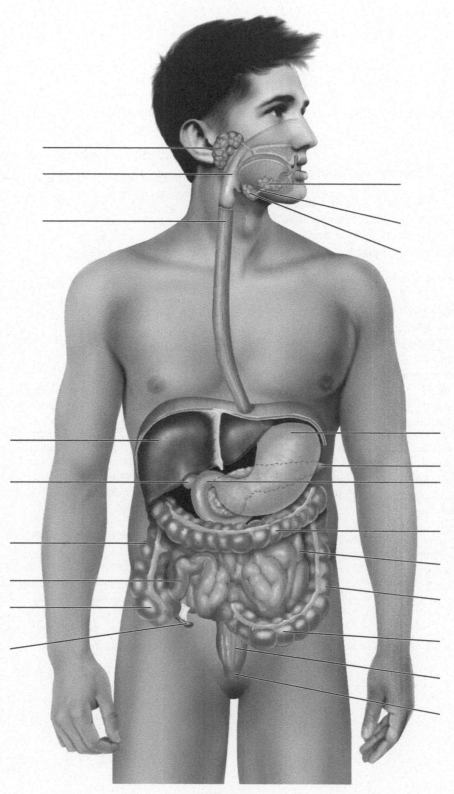

Figure 15-2

Select the correct answer.

1. Which of the following is a function of nutrients in the body?
   a. building blocks to make new cells and tissues
   b. making the chemical compounds needed for metabolism
   c. the energy source needed to run the machinery of the body
   d. all of the above

2. What are the sequential steps in digesting, or processing, food?
   a. ingestion, digestion, absorption, and elimination
   b. ingestion, absorption, nutrition, and elimination
   c. digestion, absorption, elimination, and nutrition
   d. ingestion, absorption, elimination, and respiration

3. Food passes from mouth to anus in the following sequence:
   a. Mouth, esophagus, stomach, liver, small intestine, large intestine, anus
   b. Mouth, pharynx, esophagus, stomach, small intestine, large intestine, anus
   c. Mouth, pharynx, esophagus, liver, stomach, intestine, anus
   d. Mouth, esophagus, pancreas, stomach, small intestine, large intestine, anus

4. Three types of accessory glands that secrete digestive juices into the digestive system are
   a. salivary glands, kidneys, and liver
   b. salivary glands, pancreas, and gall bladder
   c. salivary glands, pancreas, and liver
   d. liver, pancreas, and gall bladder

5. Important folds of the peritoneum include the
   a. greater omentum
   b. lesser mesentery
   c. mesocolon
   d. a and c

6. All of the following are parts of the teeth *except*
   a. dentin
   b. crown
   c. uvula
   d. pulp

7. The _____ glands become infected and swollen as a result of some infections, including mumps (a viral infection).
   a. parotid
   b. submandibular
   c. sublingual
   d. none of the above

8. Saliva helps the tongue convert the mouthful of food to a semisolid mass called a _____, which can be easily swallowed.
   a. molecule
   b. bolus
   c. capsule
   d. uvula

9. The _____ keeps food from entering the respiratory passageways.
   a. larynx
   b. epiglottis
   c. uvula
   d. tongue

10. In gastroesophageal reflux disease (GERD), gastric juice spurts up into the esophagus causing irritation and spasms when the _____ fails to constrict completely.
    a. epiglottis
    b. pyloric sphincter
    c. cardiac sphincter
    d. duodenum

11. Which of the following is not a characteristic of the stomach?
    a. many folds called rugae
    b. simple epithelium lining that secretes large amounts of mucus
    c. millions of tiny fingerlike projections, called villi
    d. millions of gastric glands extending deep into the stomach wall

12. Most digestion takes place in the _____ of the small intestine.
    a. duodenum
    b. jejunum
    c. ileum
    d. none of the above

Mark each statement true or false; correct the false statements to make them true.

13. _____ The pancreas is both an endocrine gland that secretes the insulin and glucagon and an exocrine gland that secretes pancreatic juice.

14. _____ If the pancreas is damaged, its ducts may become blocked resulting in a condition called acute pancreatitis in which the pancreas may be digested by its own enzymes.

15. _____ The liver receives oxygen-rich blood from the hepatic portal vein and nutrient-rich blood from the hepatic arteries.

16. _____ A single liver cell can carry on more than 500 separate metabolic activities including the production of bile and the conversion of glucose to glycogen.

17. _____ In the mouth, the enzyme salivary amylase begins breaking down long glucose chains into smaller compounds, and then to the sugar maltose.

18. _____ Digestion of fat takes place mainly in the stomach where bile emulsifies fat by a detergent action that breaks large fat droplets down into smaller droplets.

19. _____ Peptides are digested by enzymes called peptidases into free amino acids, the products of protein digestion.

20. _____ Neural messages sent to the brain by way of sympathetic and parasympathetic nerves help regulate digestion.

21. _____ A villus contains a network of capillaries that branches from a venule and empties into an artery; each villus also has a central lymph node.

22. _____ Inflammation of the appendix, a tube hanging down from the end of the cecum, is known as appendicitis and can lead to peritonitis.

23. _____ A complex community of trillions of bacteria, part of the body's microbiome, live in the large intestine and are our mutualistic partners.

24. _____ An individual's total metabolic rate is the sum of the BMR (the body's basic cost of living) and the food consumed each day.

25. _____ Malnutrition may be undernutrition or overnutrition; both conditions are serious health problems for millions of people.

PART 3: ACCEPT THE CHALLENGE

1. Why does mechanical digestion begin before chemical digestion?

2. Why is consumption of foods containing cellulose important to our digestion and health?

3. In addition to the damage from obesity, why is it a health problem to substitute unhealthy foods for nutritious foods?

Answer the questions to complete the crossword puzzle.

Digest This

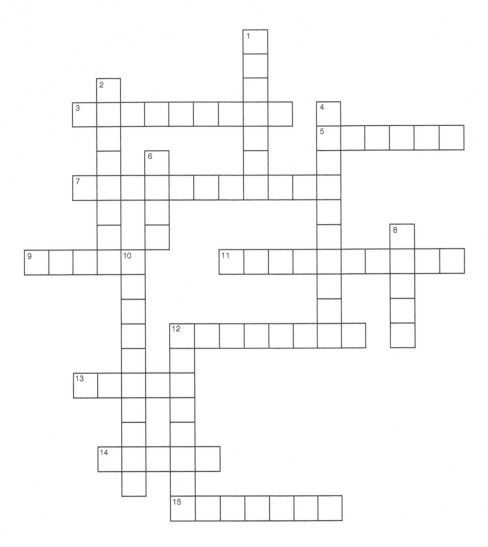

Across

3. substances in food that the body uses
5. chemical catalyst, typically a specific protein
7. reflex contractions of muscles to move food
9. soupy mixture of converted food
11. all microorganisms that live on or in body
12. consist of amino acid subunits
13. tooth area above the gum
14. largest organ; has many metabolic functions
15. large muscular organ that churns food

Down

1. central lymph vessel in villus
2. most digestion takes place here
4. enzyme that begins digestion of proteins
6. stored in the gallbladder
8. starch digestion begins here
10. flap of tissue preventing food from entering respiratory passageways
12. an endocrine and an exocrine gland

16 The Urinary System and Fluid Balance

LEARNING OBJECTIVES

1. Identify the principal metabolic waste products and the organs that excrete them.
2. Summarize the functions of the urinary system in maintaining homeostasis.
3. Describe the anatomy of the urinary system and give the function of each of its structures; label a diagram of the urinary system.
4. Connect the main structures of a nephron with their functions; label a diagram of a nephron.
5. Trace a drop of filtrate from glomerulus to urethra, listing in sequence each structure through which it passes.
6. Describe the three processes involved in urine production.
7. Describe the normal composition of urine.
8. Describe how the body regulates urine volume; include the actions of each of the hormones involved.
9. Identify the fluid compartments of the body.
10. Summarize the mechanisms that regulate fluid intake and fluid output.
11. Define electrolyte balance and summarize the functions and regulation of the major electrolytes.
12. Describe the mechanisms that maintain acid-base balance and identify causes of acidosis and alkalosis.

Match the following terms to the correct definitions by writing the corresponding letter in the space provided.
(Sections I, II)

A. elimination	B. erythropoietin	C. excretion	D. kidneys	E. nitrogenous wastes
F. renin	G. sweat glands	H. uric acid	I. urinary system	J. urine

1. _____ fluid containing water, nitrogenous wastes, and salts produced and excreted by the kidneys

2. _____ metabolic wastes that contain nitrogen

3. _____ helps regulate the volume and composition of body fluids

4. _____ discharge from the body of metabolic waste products and excess solutes

5. _____ principal organs of the urinary system

6. _____ discharge of undigested or unabsorbed food from the digestive tract

7. _____ hormone that regulates production of red blood cells

8. _____ formed from the breakdown of nucleic acids

9. _____ excrete 5% to 10% of all metabolic wastes

10. _____ enzyme important in regulating blood pressure

Fill in the blanks with the correct answer for each statement. (Section III)

11. The _____ remove metabolic wastes, excess water, and salts from the blood and produce urine, which

    passes through the paired _____ to the urinary bladder.

12. The single _____ temporarily stores urine until it is discharged from the body through the single
    urethra.

13. The kidneys, dark red and fist-sized, are located behind the _____ lining the abdominal cavity and so

    are described as retroperitoneal; they are just below the _____ and protected by the lower ribs.

14. Each kidney receives blood from a _____ and is drained by a renal vein; the ureters and blood vessels

    connect with the kidney at its _____, the notch on its medial border.

15. The kidney is covered by the _____, a tough casing of fibrous connective tissue; the kidney consists of

    an outer renal cortex and an inner _____.

16. The tip of each renal pyramid is called a _____; each renal papilla has several pores, the openings of

    _____

17. Urine passes from each collecting duct through a renal papilla and into a small tube called a _____;

    several minor calyces unite to form a _____.

18. As urine is produced, it flows into the _____, a large cavity formed by major calyces; from the renal

    pelvis, urine passes into the _____.

Match the term on the left to the correct selection on the right. (Section III)

19. _____ renal tubule

20. _____ Bowman's capsule

21. _____ nephron

22. _____ efferent arteriole

23. _____ glomerulus

24. _____ proximal convoluted tubule

25. _____ renal corpuscle

26. _____ filtrate

27. _____ peritubular capillaries

28. _____ afferent arteriole

29. _____ distal convoluted tubule

30. _____ loop of Henle

A. cluster of capillaries in the renal corpuscle

B. blood is filtered in this part of nephron

C. transports blood into the glomerulus

D. filtered fluid from renal corpuscle

E. they surround the renal tubule

F. filtrate flows here after leaving the proximal convoluted tubule

G. carries blood from glomerulus to peritubular capillaries

H. cuplike structure surrounding glomerulus

I. microscopic unit that filters blood and produces urine

J. long, partially coiled tube part of a nephron

K. coiled first part of the renal tubule

L. filtrate enters here from the loop of Henle

Fill in the blanks with the correct answer for each statement. (Section III)

31. Part of the distal convoluted tubule curves upward and contacts the afferent arteriole forming the

    _____ which secretes the enzyme renin, important in regulating blood pressure.

32. _____ passes from the kidneys into the paired ureters, ducts about 25 cm long, and is forced through

    the ureter by _____ contractions.

33. The ureters deliver urine to the _____, a temporary storage sac lined with a mucous membrane

    containing folds called rugae; the lining and _____ in the bladder wall permit it to stretch to hold up to
    800 ml of urine.

34. Urine leaves the bladder and flows through the _____, a duct leading to the outside of the body.

35. In the male, the urethra is long, passing through the _____ and the penis; in the female, the urethra is

    shorter and opens to the outside just above the opening into the _____

36. Urination, also called _____, is the process of emptying the bladder and expelling urine;

    _____ in the bladder wall are stimulated when urine volume reaches about 300 ml.

37. The receptors send a neural message to the sacral region of the spinal cord, initiating a _____, which

    contracts smooth muscle fibers in the bladder wall relaxing the _____, a ring of smooth muscle at the
    upper end of the urethra.

38. These combined actions stimulate a conscious desire to _____; the external urethral sphincter,

    composed of _____, is voluntarily relaxed and urination occurs.

39. Most young children learn to control urination by 3 years of age when the _____ has sufficiently
    matured.

Chapter **16** **The Urinary System and Fluid Balance**

Unscramble each term and match it to its correct description. (Section IV)

40. lurgralome tlifrnoati   A. substances actively transported from the blood in peritubular capillaries into filtrate in the renal tubules

41. blrtuua ptiresoronba   B. consists of blood plasma containing ions and small dissolved molecules

42. nurie   C. returns about 99% of filtrate to the blood; a highly selective process

43. utblrau cetserneio   D. important homeostatic mechanism for regulating the pH

44. ynhgdroe ino stinecreo   E. blood flows through glomerular capillaries under high pressure

45. morurglela ilraetft   F. composed of about 96% water, 2.5% nitrogen waste, 1.5% salts, and traces of other substances

Fill in the blanks with the correct answer for each statement. (Section V)

46. The body maintains a steady volume of blood and other body fluids by regulating urine volume and

_____.

47. When fluid intake is low, the body begins to _____; the concentration of dissolved salts increases as the volume of the blood _____.

48. As the blood salt concentration increases, the osmotic pressure of the blood _____.

49. When stimulated, specialized receptors in the _____ signal the posterior lobe of the pituitary gland to release _____.

50. Antidiuretic hormone (ADH) transmits information from the brain to the _____ and collecting ducts of the kidneys and makes the walls of these ducts much more permeable to water, so more water is _____ into the blood.

51. Blood volume increases, and _____ of the fluid volume is restored; a small amount of _____ urine is produced.

52. When a large amount of fluid is consumed, blood becomes diluted and its _____ falls; the _____ releases less ADH.

53. Less ADH reduces the amount of water _____ from the distal tubules and collecting ducts; a large volume of _____ urine is produced.

54. Diabetes insipidus may be diagnosed when the _____ does not produce enough ADH; _____ is not efficiently reabsorbed from the ducts resulting in the production of a large volume of urine.

55. _____, contained in coffee, tea, and alcoholic beverages, inhibits reabsorption of water, which _____ urine volume.

Match the following terms to the correct definitions by writing the corresponding letter in the space provided.
(Section V)

A. **angiotensin-converting enzyme (ACE)** B. **ACE inhibitors** C. **adrenal cortex**
D. **aldosterone** E. **angiotensin I** F. **angiotensin II**
G. **antagonistically** H. **atrial natriuretic peptide (ANP)** I. **juxtaglomerular apparatus**
J. **urine**

56. _____ renin acts on plasma protein converting it to this prehormone

57. _____ aldosterone action results in a lower volume of this

58. _____ regulates salt excretion

59. _____ cells of this secrete renin when blood pressure falls

60. _____ hormone product of the renin-angiotensin-aldosterone pathway

61. _____ converts angiotensin I into its active form (angiotensin II)

62. _____ secretes aldosterone

63. _____ block the production of angiotensin II; used to reduce hypertension

64. _____ hormone increases sodium excretion and decreases blood pressure

65. _____ renin-angiotensin-aldosterone system and ANP work this way in regulating fluid balance, salt (electrolyte) balance, and blood pressure

Fill in the blanks with the correct answer for each statement. (Section VI)

66. All of the chemical reactions in the body take place in _____, which transports materials throughout the body; it serves as an important solvent and is an essential part of many _____ reactions.

67. A solvent is the dissolving agent of a _____, and the substances dissolved in a solution are called

    _____.

68. _____ is the water in the body and the substances dissolved in it; body fluid includes the fluid inside

    cells, _____, lymph, and interstitial fluid (tissue fluid).

69. Body fluid is distributed in two principal compartments: the intracellular compartment and the _____ compartment.

70. About two-thirds of the body fluid is found in the intracellular compartment in cells and is called

    _____.

71. The remaining one-third, located outside cells in the extracellular compartment, is extracellular fluid, which

    includes _____, blood plasma and lymph, and fluid in special compartments.

72. The movement of fluid from one compartment to another depends on _____ and osmotic concentration.

73. Fluid is excreted by the kidneys and is lost through the skin, lungs, and _____; when fluid output is

    greater than fluid intake, _____ occurs.

74. Dehydration increases the osmotic pressure of the blood stimulating the thirst center in the _____; this results in the sensation of thirst and the desire to drink fluids.

Match the term on the left to the correct selection on the right. (Section VI)

75. _____ active transport

76. _____ sodium ions

77. _____ calcium ions

78. _____ phosphate ions

79. _____ anions

80. _____ ions

81. _____ electrolyte balance

82. _____ electrolytes

83. _____ cations

84. _____ potassium ions

85. _____ magnesium ions

86. _____ chloride ions

A. general term for negatively charged ions

B. electrolytes taken into the body equal to the amount lost

C. electrically charged particles

D. important in nervous and muscle tissue function, and in maintaining fluid volume within cells

E. compounds such as inorganic salts, acids, and bases that form ions in solution

F. general term for positively charged ions

G. found mainly in intracellular fluid and bone; important in the development of bones and teeth

H. needed to transmit impulses in neurons and muscle fibers

I. cells pumping specific kinds of ions into or out of each cell

J. important cation component of bones and teeth; clotting

K. help regulate differences in osmotic pressure between fluid compartments

L. most abundant intracellular ions; needed to make ATP, DNA, and RNA

Fill in the blanks with the correct answer for each statement. (Section VII)

87. Acid-base homeostasis depends on _____ concentration (pH), measured by the hydrogen ion concentration of a solution.

88. Lower pH values reflect a higher hydrogen ion concentration and indicate a stronger _____, whereas higher pH values indicate a lower hydrogen ion concentration and greater _____ (more basic).

89. Blood is slightly _____, about pH 7.4; small changes in hydrogen ion concentration can dramatically affect the distribution of other ions and can affect the rate of _____ and the structure and function of proteins.

90. A _____ is a substance that minimizes changes in pH when an acid or base is added to a solution; the main buffering systems in the body are the _____ buffer system, the phosphate buffer system, and the protein buffer systems.

91. _____ refers to any condition in which the hydrogen ion concentration of plasma is elevated above the homeostatic range; acidosis depresses the transmission of _____ across synapses.

92. _____ acidosis develops when carbon dioxide is produced more rapidly than it is excreted by the lungs.

93. _____ acidosis refers to any acidosis that is not caused by the respiratory system such as excessive exercise, causing a large accumulation of _____, or severe diarrhea from loss of bicarbonate ions.

94. _____ is any condition in which the hydrogen ion concentration is below the homeostatic range.

95. Respiratory alkalosis occurs when the respiratory system excretes _____ more quickly than it is

produced, such as during _____.

96. Excessive vomiting can lead to _____ alkalosis because hydrogen ions (from hydrochloric acid) are lost from the stomach.

97. Label the parts of the urinary system in Figure 16-1.

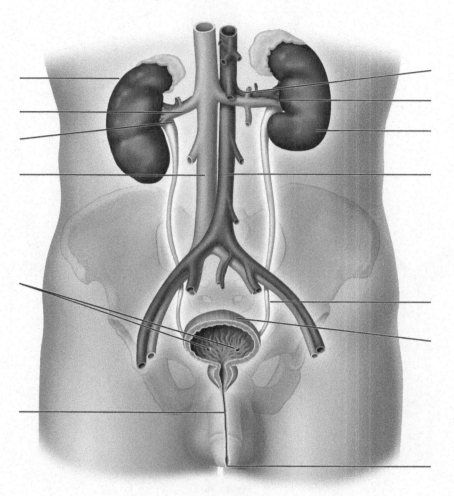

Figure 16-1

98. Label the parts of a nephron in Figure 16-2.

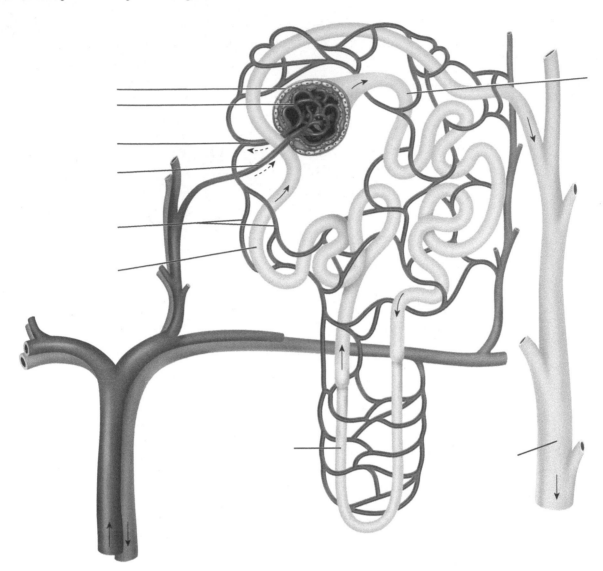

Figure 16-2

Select the correct answer.

1. Which of the following are metabolic waste products?
   a. water and glucose
   b. glucose and carbon dioxide
   c. urea and water
   d. all of the above

2. Which function is *not* performed by the urinary system?
   a. secretes the enzyme renin
   b. regulates acid-base (pH) level of the blood
   c. secretes human growth hormone
   d. regulates the quantity and concentrations of most electrolytes

3. Organs of the urinary system include all of the following *except*
   a. liver
   b. kidneys
   c. urethra
   d. ureters

4. Which of the following does *not* describe the location of the kidneys?:
   a. behind the lower ribs
   b. located near the posterior body wall
   c. located behind the peritoneum lining the abdominal cavity
   d. above diaphragm

5. Urine moves through these structures in the following sequence
   a. urethra, renal papilla, minor calyx, major calyx, renal pelvis, ureter
   b. collecting duct, renal papilla, minor calyx, major calyx, renal pelvis, ureter
   c. collecting duct, renal papilla, major calyx, renal pelvis, ureter
   d. renal papilla, major calyx, renal pelvis, ureter, urethra

6. Each renal corpuscle consists of
   a. glomerulus and renal artery
   b. glomerulus and Bowman's capsule
   c. renal tubule and Bowman's capsule
   d. renal tubule and renal artery

7. Filtrate flows in sequence through the following structures
   a. Bowman's capsule, loop of Henle, proximal convoluted tubule loop of Henle, distal convoluted tubule, and collecting duct
   b. loop of Henle, distal convoluted tubule, proximal convoluted tubule, and collecting duct
   c. Bowman's capsule, proximal convoluted tubule, loop of Henle, distal convoluted tubule, and collecting duct
   d. Bowman's capsule, distal convoluted tubule, loop of Henle, proximal convoluted tubule, and collecting duct

8. The lining and smooth muscle in the wall of the bladder allow it to stretch to hold up to

   _____ of urine.
   a. 800 ml
   b. 100 ml
   c. 500 ml
   d. 50 ml

9. The urination reflex contracts smooth muscle fibers

   in the _____ wall and also relaxes the

   _____.
   a. urethra; bladder
   b. bladder; ureters
   c. kidney; bladder
   d. bladder; internal urethral sphincter

10. Urine production involves all of the following *except*
    a. electrolyte transfer
    b. glomerular filtration
    c. tubular reabsorption
    d. tubular secretion

11. The adjusted filtrate, called urine, is composed of about
    a. 96% nitrogen wastes and 2.5% water
    b. 96% water and 2.5% nitrogen wastes
    c. 50% water and 50% nitrogenous wastes
    d. 50% electrolytes and 50% nitrogenous wastes

12. Which of the following is *not* true concerning aldosterone?
    a. produced in the hypothalamus
    b. stored in the posterior pituitary gland
    c. makes the walls of collecting ducts more permeable to water
    d. all of the above

Mark each statement true or false; correct the false statements to make them true.

13. _____ Bladder infections are more common in males than in females because the long female urethra is a barrier to bacterial invasion.

14. _____ If the urinary bladder becomes too full, urination may occur despite conscious inhibition.

15. _____ By regulating urine volume and composition, the body maintains a steady volume of blood and other body fluids.

16. _____ When the pituitary gland does not produce enough ADH, water is not efficiently reabsorbed from the collecting ducts resulting in the production of a large volume of urine, a condition called diabetes insipidus.

17. _____ When blood pressure falls, cells of the urinary bladder secrete the enzyme renin, activating the renin-angiotensin-aldosterone pathway.

18. _____ Angiotensin II constricts blood vessels and stimulates aldosterone secretion, aldosterone increases sodium reabsorption, smaller volume of urine excreted , blood pressure rises.

19. _____ The renin-angiotensin-aldosterone system and ANP work together in regulating fluid balance, salt (electrolyte) balance, and blood pressure.

20. _____ The movement of fluid from one compartment to another depends on blood pressure and osmotic concentration.

21. _____ Dehydration raises the osmotic pressure of the blood stimulating the thirst center in the hypothalamus.

22. _____ Positively charged ions are referred to as anions; negatively charged ions are cations.

23. _____ A chemical buffer is a substance that minimizes changes in pH when an electrolyte is added to a solution.

24. _____ Respiratory acidosis develops when carbon dioxide is produced more rapidly than it is excreted by the lungs.

PART 3: ACCEPT THE CHALLENGE

1. Why is it important to have urine analyzed as part of a health examination?

2. What might a reduction in urine production and darkly colored urine indicate?

3. Common ingredients in many sports drinks/beverages include water, sugar, table salt, calcium, carbohydrates, sodium, potassium, chloride, magnesium, high fructose corn syrup, artificial colors, glucose, fructose, caffeine, and artificial flavors. Which of these ingredients are electrolytes?

Find and circle the following words from Chapter 16. Words may be found from top to bottom, bottom to top, right to left, left to right, and diagonally.

```
F J L O G D K L X W F I S E N I R U X J N D M L T Q G N E X
P R P U H M O M X Z D E D P P C N U M F O T W L H J E Y P R
C P G T E D A T T O Q V R U A S J L C W I H P E B N P I W T
G N N K C V D H A F C U U S U R L N R W T Y T T G K X H Z M
R V H A E L W K P U Q Y U L V A Q P T H I D G A Z E U S M G
R V G D L N D N N Q L Z I G F P E C L F R U A A E D G E D M
A F X Z I H P W P U J H U J Y L V A R C U P X E A E R U C E
B I D E M F I K J N Z K N A T C W K Y I T E I I P F I N I H
A L I O I C M P F R U Q D F F C R S E M C W B W X L B I H T
S T M E N B V E L J G X A O O U E U C L I Y V E D I C N G G
Z R R H A G M C U Q F Q U Q B B N C R E M W V Y A I W E W O
Z A G R T F M S Y W Z N Y V E N I L A K L A D D L A T R N D
G T P U I K N R K Q Z H O O I U H Q G Z O C A D C W H F J J
Y E Y M O H P G T D X E V Y L J M T D V L L E S O C U L G V
C Q X F N S V M A F G V A E F H H V P B A O F V N S G B N J
X Z W U B O T G J L P V J W N S J B A R H T E R U C T Y R U
Y I B V V V B W O K M V L L P O O Z J X K A S T W M F E Z O
R Y Y I U Y B M X U N S X L E M R H Q X Y E Y J B J J T V E
E H I J H Y E J H I D F A A B P U E B B Z N K A C I D Y P M
D K V K U R W V F U A P C L A Y D V T F N Y M Q B O F L V R
D I U E U H Y P O T H A L A M U S S L S Q D H C Z G Y O G A
A A V L F L T I G A X H N N M I D T F U O D C A B W N R Q B
L U U V S W C S I D S E I E O Z S M A P T D N F L D S T A J
B S M D Y L M Z A E C X Y C N Z R L C J R K L P O Q E C C Q
U X F B E B X B M L E Z Z G I Z D I W C N Y V A O A C E G R
P W J T N A C P X H Q Y H R A M U Y L U E L X M R J B L B J
Y B M F D U B B E U D G K A P C B W U N T S L N W M M E K V
Q M F O I P T T K U W O O E X C R E T I O N Z W A A L D B K
X Q D R K P Q P B C B Z U P G J F Z C P T Z F J A B K A M N
D W M U Z F L R W N W X O Q N U Z S V E J Q F O Z F P L I B
```

Acid	Glomerulus
Aldosterone	Glucose
Alkaline	Hilus
Ammonia	Hypothalamus
Bladder	Kidneys
Blood	Micturition
Electrolyte	Renin
Elimination	Urea
Excretion	Urethra
Filtrate	Urine

17 Reproduction

CHAPTER GUIDE

I. The male produces sperm
  A. The testes produce sperm and hormones
  B. The conducting tubes transport sperm
  C. The accessory glands produce semen
  D. The penis delivers sperm into the female reproductive tract
  E. Hormones regulate male reproduction
II. The female produces ova and incubates the embryo
  A. The ovaries produce ova and hormones
  B. The uterine tubes transport ova
  C. The uterus incubates the embryo
  D. The vagina functions in sexual intercourse, menstruation, and birth
  E. The external genital structures are the vulva
  F. The breasts contain the mammary glands

G. Hormones regulate female reproduction
  1. The preovulatory phase consists of the first 2 weeks of the menstrual cycle
  2. The corpus luteum develops during the postovulatory phase
  3. The menstrual cycle stops at menopause
III. Fertilization is the fusion of sperm and secondary oocyte
IV. The zygote gives rise to the new individual
  A. The embryo develops in the wall of the uterus
  B. Prenatal development requires about 266 days
  C. The birth process includes labor and delivery
  D. Multiple births may be fraternal or identical
V. The human life cycle extends from fertilization to death

LEARNING OBJECTIVES

1. Connect the structures of the male reproductive system with their functions.
2. Trace the passage of sperm cells from the tubules in the testes through the conducting tubes and to ejaculation from the body in semen.
3. Compare the actions of gonadotropic hormones with the actions of testosterone in regulating male reproduction.
4. Connect the structures of the female reproductive system with their functions.
5. Trace the development of an ovum and its passage through the female reproductive system.

6. Describe the principal events of the menstrual cycle and summarize the interactions of the hormones that regulate female reproduction.
7. Describe the process of fertilization.
8. Summarize the course of development from fertilization to birth.
9. Describe the functions of the amnion and placenta.
10. Describe the three stages of the birth process.
11. List the stages of human development from embryo to old age.

PART 1: LEARN THE TERMS

Match the following terms to the correct definitions by writing the corresponding letter in the space provided. (Section I)

A. gametes
E. meiosis
 I. spermatic cord
M. spermatozoa

B. gonads
F. ovum
J. spermatocyte
N. testes

C. haploid
G. scrotum
K. spermatogenesis

D. inguinal canals
H. seminiferous
L. spermatogonia

1. _____ sperm cells

2. _____ has the normal diploid number of 46 chromosomes (23 pairs)

3. _____ sex glands

4. _____ total number of chromosomes reduced to 23 chromosomes, one-half the normal number

5. _____ stem cells located in the outer layer of seminiferous tubules

6. _____ eggs and sperm

7. _____ process of sperm production

8. _____ paired male gonads

9. _____ two nuclear and two cell divisions take place

10. _____ tubules that produce sperm cells and male hormones

11. _____ skin-covered bag suspended from the groin that holds testes

12. _____ arteries, veins, nerves, conducting tubes, and surrounding tissue attached to testes

13. _____ passageways connecting the scrotal and abdominal cavities

14. _____ female egg cell

Fill in the blanks with the correct answer for each statement. (Section I)

15. Sperm pass from the tubules inside the testes into the _____, a large, coiled tube located within the scrotum.

16. Each epididymis empties into a straight tube, the _____, or sperm duct, which passes from the scrotum through the inguinal canal as part of the _____.

17. The vas deferens is joined by the duct from each of the paired seminal vesicles to form the _____, which passes through the prostate gland and opens into the _____.

18. The single urethra, which conducts both urine and semen, passes through the _____ to the outside of the body.

19. Semen, a thick, whitish fluid, consists of _____, suspended in secretions of the accessory glands: the seminal vesicles, _____, and bulbourethral glands.

20. The paired _____ are saclike glands that secrete a thick fluid containing the sugar fructose that provides energy for the sperm cells.

21. The single _____ surrounds the urethra as the urethra emerges from the urinary bladder; the prostate gland produces a thin, alkaline secretion that neutralizes the acid secretions of the _____ making the environment more compatible for sperm.

22. The two pea-sized, _____ (also called Cowper's glands) are on each side of the urethra; these glands release an alkaline mucus secretion that lubricates the penis and helps neutralize the _____ of both the urethra and vagina.

23. During _____, the penis discharges about 2 to 4 ml of semen consisting of about 40 million sperm cells suspended in accessory gland secretions; sperm cells account for less than 1% of the total _____ volume.

Match the term on the left to the correct selection on the right. (Section I)

24. _____ androgens

25. _____ circumcision

26. _____ penis

27. _____ corpus

28. _____ erectile tissue

29. _____ prepuce

30. _____ interstitial cells

31. _____ reflex

32. _____ glans

33. _____ testosterone

A. one of three cylinders of spongy tissue under the skin of the penis

B. erection and ejaculation are this type of action

C. loose-fitting skin covering the proximal portion of glans; foreskin

D. lie between tubules in the testes, produce testosterone

E. male hormones

F. expanded tip at the end of the penis

G. hormone responsible for development of both primary and secondary male sex characteristics

H. male copulatory organ, delivers sperm into the female reproductive tract during sexual intercourse

I. common procedure performed on the penis of male babies for hygienic or religious reasons

J. contains blood vessels called sinusoids that fill with blood upon sexual stimulation

Fill in the blanks with the correct answer for each statement. (Section I)

34. _____ sex characteristics include the growth and activity of reproductive structures, including the penis and scrotum.

35. Secondary sex characteristics include deepening of the voice, _____ development, and growth of pubic, facial, and underarm hair.

36. _____ stimulates the adolescent growth spurt and oil glands in the skin.

37. The _____, at the onset of puberty, begins to secrete gonadotropin-releasing hormone (GnRH) that stimulates the anterior lobe of the pituitary gland to secrete gonadotropic hormones.

38. The gonadotropic hormones are follicle-stimulating hormone (FSH) and _____ hormone (LH).

39. _____, the period of sexual maturation, typically begins between ages 10 and 12 years and continues until ages 16 to 18 years for boys; the first sign of male puberty is typically enlargement of the _____.

40. The concentration of reproductive hormones are regulated by _____ feedback mechanisms.

41. Testosterone inhibits mainly LH secretion by acting on the _____, decreasing its secretion of GnRH; less GnRH results in _____ FSH and LH release by the pituitary.

42. Testosterone also directly _____ the anterior lobe of the pituitary by blocking the normal actions of GnRH on LH synthesis and release.

43. Label the parts of the male reproductive system in Figure 17-1.

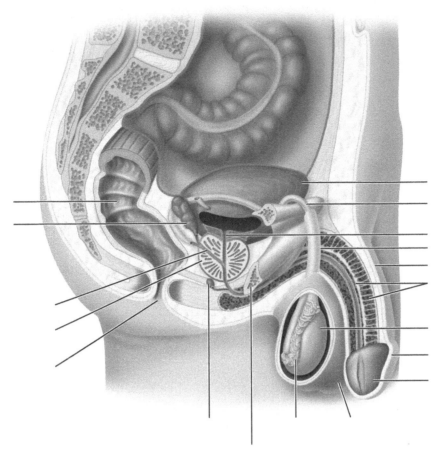

Figure 17-1

Match the following terms to the correct definitions by writing the corresponding letter in the space provided. (Section II)

A. corpus luteum   B. estrogen   C. follicle   D. oogenesis   E. oogonia
F. ovum   G. ovaries   H. ovarian ligament   I. ovulation   J. primary oocyte
K. uterine tube   L. vagina

44. _____ egg produced by females

45. _____ receives the penis and serves as the birth canal

46. _____ anchors the medial end of the ovary to the uterus

47. _____ divides to produce one secondary oocyte and one polar body during meiosis

48. _____ female gonads; produce ova and female sex hormones

49. _____ development process of ovum involving meiosis

50. _____ part of the follicle that remains behind; temporary endocrine structure

51. _____ female hormone secreted by follicles

52. _____ produced by stem cells of ovaries

53. _____ oviduct or fallopian tube

54. _____ developing ovum and its surrounding sac

55. _____ developing ovum is ejected through the wall of the ovary and into the pelvic cavity

Fill in the blanks with the correct answer for each statement. (Section II)

56. The free end of the uterine tube is funnel-shaped and has long, finger-like projections called _____;

at ovulation, the secondary oocyte is released into the _____ and drawn into the uterine tube by the beating action of the fimbriae.

57. Normally, _____ takes place in the upper one-third of the uterine tube as the fertilized egg, or

_____, begins its development as it is moved along toward the uterus.

58. The uterus prepares for a potential _____ each month during a woman's reproductive life; when

pregnancy occurs, the uterus serves as the incubator for the developing _____.

59. The tiny embryo implants itself in the _____ and develops there until it is able to live independently;

when labor occurs the uterine wall _____ powerfully and rhythmically, expelling the new baby from the mother's body.

60. If pregnancy does not occur, the inner lining of the uterus sloughs off and is discarded in a process called

_____, which occurs every month.

61. The _____ is a hollow, pear-shaped organ about the size of a small fist at its widest region; it lies

in the bottom of the pelvic cavity, anterior to the rectum and posterior to the _____.

62. The main portion of the uterus is the _____, or body; the rounded part of the uterus above the level of

the entering uterine tubes is the _____.

63. The lower, narrow portion of the uterus is the _____, which partially projects into the vagina; cervical cancer is a common type of cancer in women that can be successfully treated when detected at very early stages

during a routine _____.

Match the term on the left to the correct selection on the right. (Section II)

64. _____ vulva

65. _____ rugae

66. _____ labia minora

67. _____ fornices

68. _____ labia majora

69. _____ hymen

70. _____ vagina

71. _____ vestibule

A. mound of fatty tissue that covers the pubic symphysis

B. recesses formed between the vaginal wall and cervix

C. contains openings of the urethra and vagina

D. diamond-shaped region between the pubic arch and anus

E. external female genital structures

F. folds of skin that pass from mons pubis to the region behind the vaginal opening

G. elastic, muscular tube that extends from the cervix to its opening to the outside of the body

H. small structure that corresponds to the male glans penis

72. _____ clitoris

73. _____ mons pubis

74. _____ Bartholin's glands

75. _____ perineum

I. folds in the vagina, which straighten out to enlarge this organ during sexual intercourse and childbirth

J. two thin folds of skin located just within labia majora

K. thin ring of mucous membrane that surrounds the entrance to the vagina

L. open on each side of the vaginal opening; secrete lubricating mucus

Unscramble each term and match it to its correct description. (Section II)

76. lotsmcoru

77. prnicalot

78. cotnxioy

79. pelnpi

80. amaymmr lgasnd

81. tatlnoaci

82. easbrt renacc

A. duct draining milk opens at the surface of this smooth muscle

B. production and release of milk for nourishment of a baby

C. located within the breasts; produce milk

D. common cancer in women; high survival rate with early diagnosis and treatment

E. secreted by anterior pituitary; stimulates milk production

F. fluid produced by mammary glands for the first few days after childbirth

G. stimulates ejection of milk from the glands into the ducts

Fill in the blanks with the correct answer for each statement. (Section II)

83. Hormones released by the hypothalamus, pituitary gland, and ovaries interact to regulate _____.

84. As puberty approaches, the _____ produces GnRH; the anterior lobe of the pituitary gland then secretes FSH and LH, which signal the _____ to begin functioning.

85. The ovaries secrete _____ and progesterone; estrogens are responsible for the primary sex characteristics, including growth of the sex organs at _____.

86. Estrogen is also responsible for the development of _____ sex characteristics, including breast development, broadening of the _____, and the fat distribution and muscle that shape the female body.

87. _____ typically begins in girls between 10 and 12 years and continues until 14 to 16 years; _____ is usually the first sign that puberty is imminent.

88. Menarche, the first _____, usually occurs between 12 and 14 years; this cycle occurs every month from puberty until _____ at about age 50 years.

89. Interaction of FSH and LH with estrogens and progesterone from the _____ regulates the menstrual cycle; estrogens stimulate the growth of follicles and stimulate thickening of the _____.

90. A menstrual cycle is approximately 28 days long with _____ typically occurring around the 14th day.

91. Menstruation occurs during approximately the first 5 days when the thickened _____ of the uterus sloughs off; during the preovulatory phase, FSH stimulates a few _____ to develop in the ovary.

92. The developing follicles release _____ stimulating endometrial growth again and redevelopment of blood vessels and glands; after the first week, typically only one follicle continues to develop.

93. _____ feedback signals from increasing estrogen concentration and inhibin, secreted by the ovary, inhibits further secretion of FSH.

94. As estrogen concentration peaks, it signals the anterior pituitary gland to secrete LH, a _____ feedback mechanism; this surge of LH stimulates final maturation of the follicle and _____.

95. The _____ phase begins after ovulation when LH stimulates development of the corpus luteum, a temporary endocrine structure that releases progesterone and estrogens; these hormones stimulate continued thickening of the endometrium, preparing for a _____.

96. The _____ begins to degenerate if pregnancy does not occur; progesterone and estrogen levels rapidly decline as small arteries in the uterine wall constrict, depriving the endometrium of _____; the small blood vessels then rupture.

97. At menopause, estrogen and progesterone secretion decreases and the female is no longer _____; the decrease in hormones can cause a variety of symptoms, including uncomfortable heat sensation (hot flashes).

98. Label the parts of the female pelvic area in Figure 17-2.

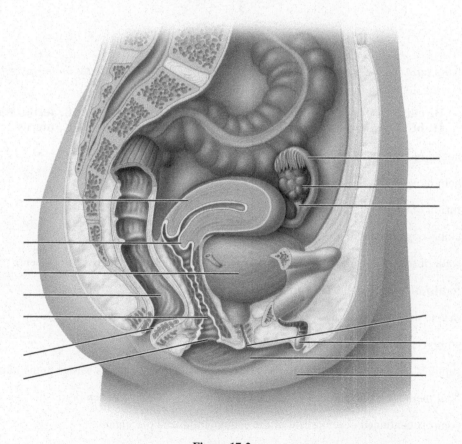

Figure 17-2

99. Label the parts of the female reproductive system in Figure 17-3.

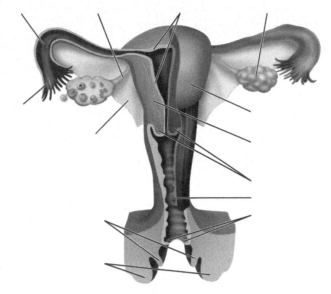

Figure 17-3

Match the following terms to the correct definitions by writing the corresponding letter in the space provided. (Section III, IV)

A. amnion	**B. cilia**	**C. conception**	**D. embryo**	**E. fertilization**	**F. fetus**
G. gestation	**H. hCG hormone**	**I. placenta**	**J. umbilical cord**	**K. uterus**	**L. zygote**

100. _____ nuclei of sperm and ovum fuse to form fertilized egg or this

101. _____ help move embryo toward the uterus

102. _____ fusion of sperm and egg

103. _____ embryo is referred to this after 8 weeks of gestation

104. _____ stalk of tissue, containing two arteries and a vein, connecting embryo with placenta

105. _____ fertilization and establishing pregnancy

106. _____ zygote divides producing two-celled

107. _____ embryo plants itself in this wall at the 7th day of development

108. _____ supplies oxygen and nutrients to the embryo; transfers the embryo's wastes to the mother's blood

109. _____ fetal membrane that forms a fluid-filled, cushioning sac around the embryo

110. _____ controls continued development of the endometrium and placenta

111. _____ period of development from conception to birth

Fill in the blanks with the correct answer for each statement. (Section IV)

112. A baby requires 38 weeks for development from _____ to delivery.

113. The brain and _____ are among the first organs to develop and by 4 weeks the eyes and ears are

    visible; a simple _____ system is working.

114. Small mounds of tissue called _____, which can be seen after the first month, slowly lengthen,
    forming the limbs.

115. By the end of the third month, the _____ is more than 6 cm long and weighs about 14 g; by 5 months

    of development, the fetus moves about in the _____ and the mother usually feels the fetal movements.

116. During the last 3 months (last trimester) growth and _____ of tissues and organs is rapid; the

    cerebrum grows rapidly, developing _____ (folds) during month seven, and most of the body
    becomes covered by downy hair (lanugo).

117. Several days before birth, the fetus typically assumes an upside-down position, which prepares it to enter the

    _____ headfirst.

118. Childbirth, or _____, includes labor and delivery; during the first stage of labor, a long series of

    involuntary uterine _____ occur.

119. The cervix becomes _____ to about 10 cm and becomes effaced, continuous with the uterine wall, so
    it cannot be distinguished from the adjoining portion of the uterus; this process allows passage of the baby's

    _____.

120. The amnion may rupture and release _____ through the vagina during the first stage of labor, which
    often lasts 8 to 24 hours in a first pregnancy.

121. The _____ begins when the cervix is fully dilated and ends with the baby's delivery; the mother helps

    push the baby through the vagina by contracting her _____ muscles.

122. When the neonate (newborn) emerges, physicians clamp and cut the _____, which separates it from

    the placenta; the placenta separates from the _____ and is expelled in the third stage of labor, usually
    within 10 to 20 minutes after the baby's birth.

123. The placenta, referred to as the _____, is inspected for abnormalities and then discarded.

Match the term on the left to the correct selection on the right. (Section IV, V)

124. _____ adolescence	A.	extends from birth to the end of the first month of postnatal life
125. _____ identical twins	B.	infancy until adolescence
126 _____ infancy	C.	dizygotic twins; two eggs are ovulated and each is fertilized by a different sperm
127. _____ fertility drugs	D.	adolescence until about age 40
128. _____ neonatal period	E.	twins arising from two masses of cells that fail to separate completely
129. _____ young adulthood	F.	begins at age 80
130. _____ childhood	G.	monozygotic twins; develop when cells that make up an early embryo divides to form two independent cell groups
131 _____ conjoined	H.	time of development between puberty and adulthood
132. _____ fraternal twins	I.	from neonatal period until age 2 years
133. _____ middle age	J.	use of these have made multiple births much more common
134. _____ old age	K.	begins at age 40

167

Select the correct answer.

1. Which event must occur first for reproduction to take place?
   a. fertilization
   b. formation of gametes
   c. sexual intercourse
   d. ejaculation

2. Reproductive functions are primarily regulated by the interactions of
   a. males and females
   b. pituitary hormones and gonads
   c. neurons and gametes
   d. growth hormones and sexual intercourse

3. Which of the following is *not* a male reproductive structure?
   a. testes
   b. prostate gland
   c. penis
   d. uterine tube

4. _____ prevents doubling of the chromosome number each time fertilization occurs.
   a. Meiosis (Reduction division)
   b. Mitosis
   c. Reproduction
   d. Fertilization

5. The spermatic cord includes
   a. arteries and veins
   b. nerves
   c. connective tissue
   d. all of the above

6. Sperm pass through the following sequence of structures
   a. epididymis, testes, vas deferens, ejaculatory duct, urethra
   b. vas deferens, seminiferous tubules in testis, epididymis, urethra
   c. seminiferous tubules in testis, epididymis, vas deferens, ejaculatory duct, urethra
   d. epididymis, testes, vas deferens, penis, urethra

7. PSA is a tumor marker because its elevation is associated with _____.
   a. penile cancer
   b. prostate cancer
   c. pituitary tumors
   d. none of the above

8. A man may be considered sterile if his semen contains less than
   a. 40 million sperm/L
   b. 20 million sperm/ml
   c. 20 billion sperm/ml
   d. 40 million sperm/ml

9. The gonadotropic hormones, secreted by the pituitary gland, are
   a. gonadotropin-releasing hormone (GnRH) and inhibin
   b. follicle-stimulating hormone (FSH) and luteinizing hormone (LH)
   c. follicle-stimulating hormone (FSH) and inhibin
   d. luteinizing hormone (LH) and testosterone

10. All of the following are female reproductive organs *except*
    a. vagina
    b. breasts
    c. perineum
    d. uterus

11. The ovaries, the female sex gonads, produce ova and the female sex hormones
    a. estrogens and progesterone
    b. progesterone and human growth hormone
    c. estrogens and gonadotropin
    d. progesterone and oxytocin

12. The process of ovum development, called oogenesis, follows this sequence
    a. Primary oocyte (diploid), oogonium (diploid), secondary oocyte + polar body (both haploid), (after fertilization) ovum + polar body (both haploid)
    b. Oogonium (diploid), primary oocyte (diploid), ovum + polar body (both haploid), (after fertilization) secondary oocyte + polar body (both haploid)
    c. Oogonium (diploid), primary oocyte (diploid), secondary oocyte + polar body (both haploid), (after fertilization) ovum + polar body (both haploid)
    d. Primary oocyte (diploid), primary oocyte (diploid), ovum + polar body (both haploid), secondary oocyte + polar body (both haploid)

13. The part of the follicle that remains behind in the ovary develops into an important temporary endocrine structure, the _____.
    a. oviduct
    b. ovum
    c. embryo
    d. corpus luteum

Mark each statement true or false; correct the false statements to make them true.

14. _____ Movements of the fimbriae and the current created by the beating of cilia in the lining of the tube draw the secondary oocyte into the uterine tube.

15. _____ Fertilization normally takes place in the upper one-third of the uterus and the fertilized egg, or zygote, begins its development as it is moved along toward the cervix.

16. _____ If pregnancy does not occur, the inner lining of the uterus sloughs off and is discarded in a process, called menopause, which occurs every month.

17. _____ The uterus is lined by the endometrium, which becomes thick and vascular and develops glands that secrete a nourishing fluid each month in preparation for possible pregnancy.

18. _____ Cervical cancer has been linked to infection with human papillomavirus (HPV); effective vaccines against HPV, available for females and males, also prevent certain other sexually transmitted diseases.

19. _____ The vagina is a stiff, muscular tube that receives the penis during sexual intercourse and provides nourishment and oxygen for the developing fetus.

20. _____ The female breast is composed of lobes of adipose tissue, which produce milk; the amount of glandular tissue around these lobes determines the size of the breasts and affects their capacity to produce milk.

21. _____ Prolactin, secreted by the anterior pituitary, stimulates the breasts to produce milk, which normally begins the third day after delivery of the baby.

22. _____ Like testosterone in the male, estrogens are responsible for the growth of sex organs at puberty (primary sex characteristics) and for the development and maintenance of secondary sex characteristics.

23. _____ Interaction of FSH and LH with estrogens and progesterone from the ovaries regulates the menstrual cycle, which occurs every month from puberty until menopause.

24. _____ During the preovulatory phase, estrogen inhibits secretion of FSH and ovarian cells secrete prostaglandin, which also inhibits FSH secretion; these positive feedback signals result in an increase in FSH concentration.

25. _____ The following occurs during fertilization: a sperm enters the ovum, the second meiotic division takes place, the nuclei of the sperm and ovum then fuse to form a fertilized egg, or zygote.

26. _____ The placenta produces hCG, which signals the corpus luteum to grow and to release large amounts of estrogen and progesterone, stimulating the endometrium and placenta to continue their development.

27. _____ Identical twins develop when two eggs are ovulated and each is fertilized by a different sperm. Each fertilized egg has its own unique genetic endowment.

1. What is the evolutionary significance of meiosis?

2. Why do males ejaculate millions of sperm when only one sperm is required for fertilization?

3. What is the disadvantage of the zygote implanting before reaching the uterine wall?

THE PUZZLE

Answer the questions to complete the crossword puzzle.

It's Reproducible

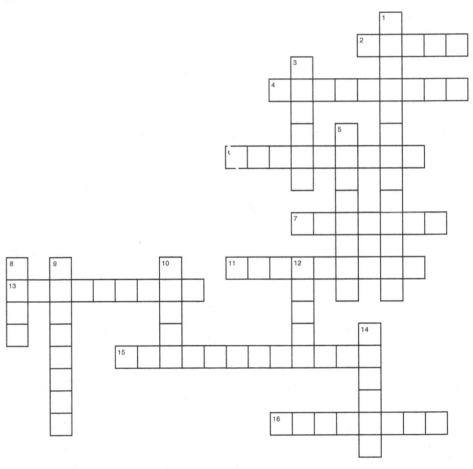

Across

2. embryo is this after 8 weeks of gestation
4. period of development from conception to birth
6. development process of ovum involving meiosis
7. skin-covered bag suspended from the groin that holds testes
11. infancy until adolescence
13. contains opening of the urethra and opening of the vagina
15. responsible for development of primary and secondary male sex characteristics
16. common cancer in women

Down

1. fusion of sperm and egg
3. erection and ejaculation are actions
5. onset of menstruation
8. female egg cell
9. hormone responsible for female sex characteristics
10. expanded tip at the end of the penis
12. begins with a long series of involuntary uterine contractions
14. becomes fully dilated at childbirth